Calisthenics:

Upper

Body

Blast

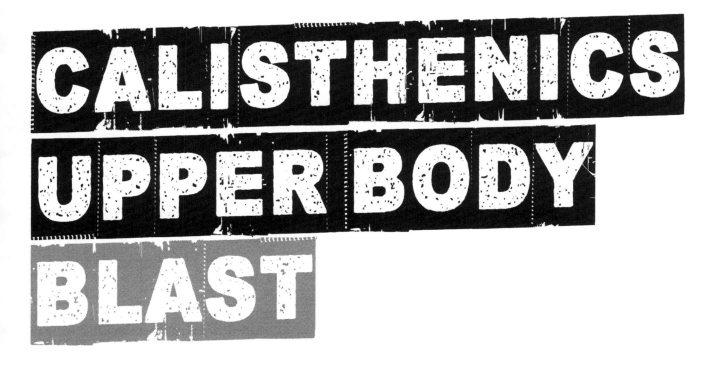

CALISTHENICS UPPER BODY BLAST

THE #1 CHEST, ARMS, SHOULDERS & BACK BODYWEIGHT TRAINING GUIDE

PURECALISTHENICS

Disclaimer:

This guide has been created for informational and reference purposes only. The author, publisher and other affiliated parties cannot be held in any way accountable for any personal injuries or damage allegedly resulting from the information contained herein, or from any misuse of such guidance. Although strict measures have been taken to provide accurate information, the parties involved with the creation and publication of this guide take no responsibility for any issues that may arise from alleged discrepancies contained herein. It is strongly recommended that you consult a physician, personal trainer and nutritionist prior to commencing this or any other workout or diet plan. This guide is not a substitute for professional personal guidance from a qualified medical professional. If you feel pain or discomfort at any point during the exercises contained herein, cease the activity immediately and seek medical guidance. This resource has been created to teach calisthenics in a progressive way, and you should not advance until you have completed the simpler exercises as recommended with perfect form. It is strongly recommended that you use a spotter or personal trainer at all times.

calisthenics

[kal-*uh* s-**then**-iks]

Noun

1. *Gymnastic exercises designed to develop physical strength, vigor and grace of movement, usually performed with little or no special apparatus.*

Origin

Greek *kallos* "beauty" + *sthenos* "strength" + -ics.

BEFORE YOU BEGIN:

BONUS GIFT: FREE CALISTHENICS TRAINING PROGRAM

As a token of gratitude for picking up this book we'd love to give you a free body-weight exercise program to help you on your way to superhuman shape!

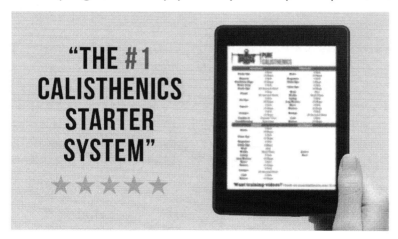

Visit **www.purecalisthenics.com** for your training program!

CONTENTS

INTRODUCTION

Congratulations, you have just invested in the world's most effective training system. This book is part of The SUPERHUMAN Series, and in this edition you will be building up your arms, chest, shoulders and back like a SPARTAN!

This guide has been designed to teach calisthenics in a progressive way, with multiple variations on popular exercises increasing in intensity and difficulty as you make your way through. Follow our guidance to the letter, adhere to the structure set out and you will experience MIND-BLOWING results.

Whether you are completely new to exercise or switching over to calisthenics from weightlifting or anything else, this book is for you. Get started now and take the first step on the path to a stronger, fitter, more powerful you.

To stay up to date with the latest trends in bodyweight exercise, please join us online at purecalisthenics.com for training tips, equipment reviews, nutrition advice and more. You can also find us on Twitter and Facebook - just search 'Pure Calisthenics'.

For more calisthenics resources, check out our full range of books by searching 'Pure Calisthenics' on Amazon. For now, it's time to get down to business. Read on, comrade, and unlock your potential with Upper Body BLAST!

Train hard!

The Pure Calisthenics Team

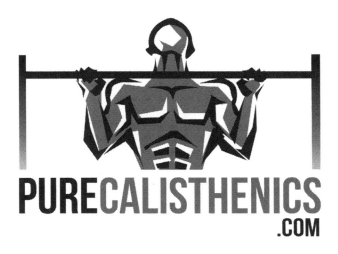

How to Use This Book

This book is your training bible. You should not merely read the words; you should LIVE by them. Yes, there will be times when you want to give up, but pressing on ahead is what separates the best from the rest.

Use these 4 quick tips to help maximize your results:

1. Prepare

Don't just dive straight into the exercises headfirst and go crazy, you will put yourself at risk of injury. Read through the introductory chapters of this book so you know exactly how to approach your training.

2. Focus

Calisthenics is not just about physical strength, but also mental fortitude. Your friends may swear by free weights and there's nothing wrong with that if they want to train isolated muscle groups. You, however, are training to achieve complete body perfection and you must stand by your decision. Don't allow anyone to influence your thinking – you are training for YOUR goals, not theirs.

3. Commit

As with any form of exercise, you need to be fully committed to a consistent workout program if you want to see results. Don't think you can simply throw in a few body-weight movements here and there and go home looking like a Greek god. Calisthenics requires you to GIVE everything if you want to TAKE everything. Follow a proper training schedule and stick to it. You'll find a link to our free program at the back of this book.

4. Think Long-Term

Following on from the above, it is important to maintain a long-term vision for your training. There is no miracle formula for a better body, but calisthenics is as close as you can get. Set realistic goals and commit to achieving them within a reasonable time frame and, in time, you will achieve incredible levels of strength and physical ability. Don't forget to keep track of your progress and celebrate the little wins along the way.

Now the pep talk is out of the way, let's move on!

1. What is Calisthenics?

If you're reading this book then the chances are you've already looked into calisthenics, probably read a few articles online and watched some videos of seemingly superhuman feats of strength by famous practitioners on YouTube.

These guys have it all; traps that reach up to their ears, sculpted shoulders, bulging chests, forearms like Popeye, abs you could grate cheese on and legs that could propel them to the moon. And all without pumping iron? Well, pretty much.

How Does it Work?

Calisthenics, by definition, is a form of exercise that consists of various gross motor movements using your own bodyweight for resistance, normally without equipment or apparatus, with the exception of basic items such as a pull-up bar or parallettes.

This is the art of training your body as nature intended; not by isolating muscle groups and using complex man-made machinery that you would never find out in the real world, but by using the tools you are already equipped with. With calisthenics, your body is your gym, and the world is your playground.

What Does it Do?

Calisthenics is the art of strengthening your entire body as a unit, eliminating each weak link in the chain until every fiber of your being is working in total harmony to produce extraordinary levels of strength.

Training like this achieves results you can use in the real world. Think about it, how often do you need to bicep curl something, or flap cables around over your head in everyday life? These are all man-made inventions designed to make single muscle groups strong IN THE GYM, but as soon as we step outside it becomes somewhat irrelevant.

To perform at maximum capacity in everyday life, or to acquire formidable strength and fitness for your sport, you need to be strong everywhere, not just in certain places.

Calisthenics strengthens every muscle group and every link between those muscle groups. It is the ultimate form of exercise for creating true strength that you can use every day, whether it be for regular tasks, your favorite sport or just showing off!

WHO IS IT FOR?

The simple answer to this question is that calisthenics is for everyone. Practicing body-weight training can help anyone achieve a stronger, fitter, more flexible body.

Whether you are a lean athlete wanting to pile on more muscle mass, a 200-pound bodybuilder seeking to get shredded, a kick boxer requiring greater range of motion or simply starting up with exercise for the first time, calisthenics is the ultimate solution.

Don't just take our word for it. Professional sports teams and global militias often utilize calisthenics for its explosive effectiveness and practical application. You can use your bodyweight to train any place, any time, making it the benchmark fitness solution for high level operators across the world.

Don't get stuck performing the same old isolated exercises in the gym for years on end, choose calisthenics and take your gym with you wherever you go!

HOW CAN I GET STARTED?

One of the great advantages of calisthenics is that it's super simple to get started. You don't need a gym membership or any prior experience, and you can begin with simple exercises today.

With that in mind, here's a few key tips to make life easier for those just getting started:

1. Use a credible guide: This is your starting point! Don't dive straight in and use guess-work to correct course, as this often ends in disappointment or, worse, injury. Whether you choose to follow this guide or something else, the most important thing is that you stick to it like glue, and let the experts guide you to success.

2. Establish a program: Training without a program is like driving around a strange place without a map. In order to stay on track and keep up to date with your progress, you need a schedule. You can get one at the back of this book, or work with a trainer to create your own.

3. Get a training partner: Tests prove that accountability is a hugely effective catalyst for increasing performance. For us, this means getting a committed training partner and supporting each other on the journey.

Above all, starting up is as simple as putting on your sweats and getting out there. So, step up and step out, companion, it all begins here!

"There are no limits. There are only plateaus, and you must not stay there, you must go beyond them."

Bruce Lee

2. DIET AND NUTRITION

We can practically hear some of you screaming, 'I know what to eat, just get to the good stuff already!'

Well, we're going to shut you down like a rat-infested restaurant right now because diet and nutrition are the foundation of a great body and it would be a dereliction of duty to neglect this area.

If you want to maximize your results then don't skip this part.

HYDRATE

Water is life. We need it to transport vital nutrients around the body and to keep our muscles and minds functioning at full capacity.

Most people simply do not drink enough water day-to-day, which means both their performance *and* their recovery is greatly impaired.

According to The European Food Safety Authority, men should be drinking about 2 liters of water per day while women should get about 1.6 liters. This is, of course, a general guideline but if you are not hitting these figures you may be affected by dehydration. We recommend speaking to a physician or nutritionist to discuss your requirements.

If you are taking a supplement such as creatine, which affects the way that your body processes water, then you will need to drink more. Check out the label on all of your supplements and always ensure you take on board enough fluids.

While we're on the topic, steer clear of alcohol and fizzy drinks if you want to get ripped. They're packed full of carbs and sugar, and won't do you any favors whatsoever.

EAT RIGHT

Your particular goals will determine your diet, but there are some general guidelines to follow here if you want to get in the best shape possible.

Eat clean: We're not asking you to become a hippy or go plucking fruits from trees, but it really pays to cut out processed food and other junk. Check the labels and pick up fresh foods which contain a single ingredient – i.e. whatever it is actually supposed to be – rather than something packed full of preservatives and lord knows what else.

Mix it up: You've heard it said over and over and now you're going to hear it once again; a balanced and varied diet is the key to good health. This means a mixture of proteins, carbohydrates and fats. Check out the following examples for some inspiration:

Proteins: Organic meat, poultry, fish, eggs and dairy are primary sources of protein.

Carbohydrates: Fruits and vegetables are a great source of healthy carbohydrates, as are sweet potatoes, wholegrain pastas, brown rice and similar grains.

Fats: Forget the myth of fat being bad for you. The type found in good quality meats, nuts, seeds, fish and olive oil is an essential part of your daily diet.

EAT FOR YOUR GOAL

When you strip diet and fitness down to their core elements it becomes very simple. If you want to gain weight and muscle mass, you simply have to eat more calories than you burn off.

If you want to maintain your weight and refine your body then you should be aiming to eat around the same amount of calories as you burn off. If you want to cut down then you should be burning off more calories than you are eating.

There are plenty of resources out there to assist you with your particular objective, but we would advise against obsessive calorie counting. Food should be something to look forward to and you will soon start to resent it if preparation becomes a chore. By all means use tools and technology to ensure you are on the right track, but don't beat yourself up over fractions of a gram.

With that said, you should be aware of your macros and make a conscious effort to meet them on a daily basis. If you're not sure what this means, it is essentially just the combination of fats, carbs and proteins which make up your diet. Everybody is different and only you can determine what is appropriate for your body and goals, but if you are unsure, it pays to contact a professional nutritionist for guidance.

Planning meals in advance and cooking in bulk is super useful here, as it cuts out the guesswork and reduces the risk of making poor decisions on impulse!

We could write a whole book on diet and nutrition, and perhaps we will, but this one is about calisthenics, so for now we must move on. Suffice it to say, though, that you should pay special attention to your diet and take the time to investigate it thoroughly in order to maximize your results.

"Looking good and feeling good go hand in hand. If you have a healthy lifestyle, your diet and nutrition are set, and you're working out, you're going to feel good."

Jason Statham

3. KNOW YOUR BODY

Think you know your body? Think again. It's one thing to isolate muscles with regular exercises such as the bench press or bicep curl but it is entirely another to employ whole groups at the same time to squeeze out that last gut-busting muscle-up or planche.

Putting yourself under such intense strain can be dangerous if you don't know what you are doing, so it is important to familiarize yourself with your body to ensure you are utilizing it correctly and not putting yourself at risk of harm.

We suggest keeping a body map handy. You'll find a basic one on the next page, but it's a good idea to take your learning further, otherwise you may have no idea what we mean when we discuss certain muscle groups.

There is no shortage of quality resources out there when it comes to biomechanics and the study of the human body, and the more you learn the more control you will have over your progress and results.

In addition to DIY textbook style studying, we always recommend hooking up with a qualified and reputable personal trainer or physician to assess your individual needs and goals, since we cannot be there to advise everyone in person.

Super important: If at any time you feel pain or discomfort during exercise, STOP. Try some slow, steady movements to test the area and stretch it out gently.

If pain persists or worsens, call it a day and seek advice on the issue. Refer back to the body map to hone in on the area and speak to a physician for further advice.

Only return to training when you can comfortably perform movements without feeling any pain or impingements. Do not be tempted to 'power through' an injury as this will only exacerbate the issue and delay your recovery time. It is much smarter to take a short break and get back on track quickly than to finish your session at the cost of weeks or even months out of action.

Remember, calisthenics may be completely different to anything you have performed before. You will likely awaken muscles you never even knew existed, and it is probably going to hurt like hell, so make sure you are suitably prepared.

To help brace your body for action we'll be covering warm-up and preparation next.

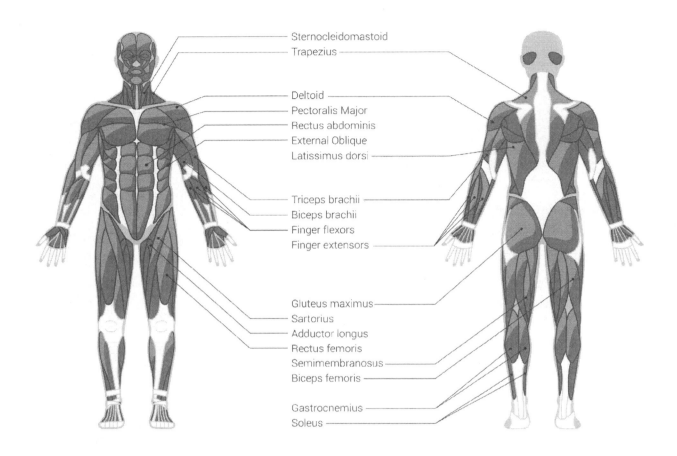

Sternocleidomastoid
Trapezius
Deltoid
Pectoralis Major
Rectus abdominis
External Oblique
Latissimus dorsi
Triceps brachii
Biceps brachii
Finger flexors
Finger extensors
Gluteus maximus
Sartorius
Adductor longus
Rectus femoris
Semimembranosus
Biceps femoris
Gastrocnemius
Soleus

Above: A basic body map showing the major muscle groups. It is possible to drill down into much more detail, but we simply do not have the scope to cover everything in this guide. We highly recommend that you take your learning as far as time allows.

Remember, although we share the same basic physiology - with the exception of the obvious differences between the male and female anatomy - every individual is unique. Genetic factors beyond our control give us the blueprint with which we must work.

Instead of trying to 'fight' your genetics, we recommend working with them in order to sculpt your perfect body. If this sounds a bit heavy, don't worry, it simply means getting to know your strengths and weaknesses and working with those, instead of trying to force yourself down a path your body isn't prepared for.

That's not to say you can't build your dream physique, only that you should take a smart and informed approach. As always, we recommend speaking to a pro for more advice.

"Success is no accident. It is hard work, perseverance, learning, studying, sacrifice and most of all, love of what you are doing or learning to do."

Pele

4. Warm-Up & Preparation

Whether you are a seasoned gym-goer or a complete newbie, calisthenics will shock your body to the core. You will awaken muscles you never even knew existed and aches and pains will spring up all over as you become stronger as a unit. For this reason it is essential to prepare properly if you want to achieve stunning results.

The benefits of warming up are threefold:

1. By getting the blood pumping and warming up your muscles you can hit the ground running and maximize performance during your workout.

2. You minimize the risk of getting injured during training, meaning you won't have to cut sessions short or drop out entirely due to niggles or tears.

3. Stretching helps you become more flexible over time, meaning you can increase your range of motion and subsequently push your body to new limits. As you scale up in this way you will gain unprecedented strength and capability.

Some people consider warming up to be a waste of time, but if you're not willing to put in an extra 5-10 minutes per session then we would have to question your commitment to calisthenics and fitness in the first place.

When you stop thinking of a warm-up as a chore and see the serious value it brings, it will revolutionize your workout and help you along the way to results you never thought were possible. But hey, don't just take our word for it.

Consider any of your favorite sports teams or stars. From professional football clubs to mixed martial artists, Olympic rowers to tennis players and everyone in-between, there is not a single person who steps out without some form of warm-up. If it's good enough for the greatest in the world, it's sure as hell good enough for us.

Remember: This book is focused on calisthenics, and while we can cover some essential mobility and flexibility exercises we simply don't have space for a complete solution. Use the following as a guideline and build your own warm-up routine over time. Add it to your routine and consider it sacred. Don't rush it, and don't skip it.

So, now that you understand the myriad of benefits warm-up and preparation brings to your workouts, let's get to work, shall we?

HANDS

In order to transfer maximum power from your hands to whatever piece of apparatus you are using you must ditch the gloves and go bare skin. This may seem somewhat counterintuitive, because many gloves do offer additional exterior grip and most will make things more comfortable. Long-term, though, they will do more harm than good.

Consider pull-ups, for example. The extra layer between your hands and the bar means you are only as strong as your grip on the inside of the gloves. It doesn't matter how sticky the outsides are, because when that inner material starts sliding around, you'll drop like a sack of spuds.

So, the only way to transfer 100% of your energy to the bar is to make a direct and true connection. Your hands are going to take a battering and might feel sore at first but over time you will condition them to cope with these stresses and ultimately reap the rewards of a vice-like grip.

If you are using chalk or liquid chalk to help with your grip you might find your hands become very dry over time. Be sure to wash it off completely once you're finished and, if necessary, use a moisturizer.

You are unlikely to tear your hands apart when you are just getting started, but if for any reason you do cut them open don't act tough and carry on as this could put you out of action for weeks. It's best to rest for a day or two and let them heal before continuing.

Calluses are to be expected, but cuts and scars are not badges of honor to be worn with pride; they are a sign of bone-headed stupidity. Take care of your hands, and they will take care of you!

CARDIOVASCULAR

Once your hand preparation is taken care of, the first port of call in your pre-workout warm-up is to raise your heart rate and get the blood pumping.

Try 5-10 minutes of the following dynamic exercises to achieve this:

• Jogging, skipping, star jumps, cross-trainer, rowing

There are plenty of other ways to get your cardio fix, so mix it up a bit each day. Don't go overboard and leave yourself keeled over in exhaustion, but make sure it is intense enough to leave you a little out of breath. Your heart should be beating faster, and a light sweat is a good sign that you are ready to move on.

MOBILITY / MOTION

You've completed phase one of your warm-up, so the blood should now be pumping around your body, letting you know that you are ready to loosen up the areas you'll be hitting in your workout. We'll now run through some gentle mobility exercises designed to loosen up your limbs and increase your range of motion.

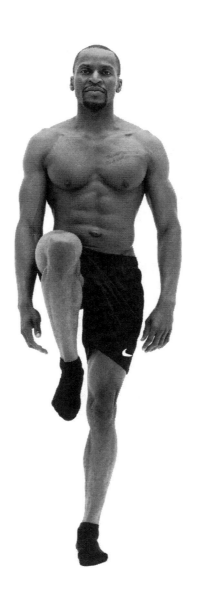

Upper Body

You will use every muscle fiber your upper body has to offer when training calisthenics so it is essential to get it ready for the task. Spend another 5-10 minutes going through the following, paying special attention to the areas of the body you plan to work out.

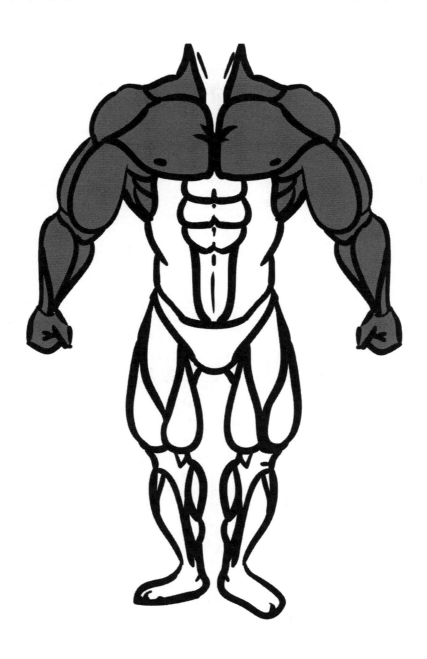

WRIST ROTATES

Your wrists are taxed in almost every calisthenics exercise, so try this simple warm-up to keep them strong and safe.

Perform: 10 seconds in each direction.

1. Extend your arms straight out in front of you.

2. Rotate your wrists clockwise for 10 seconds.

3. Switch directions and go again.

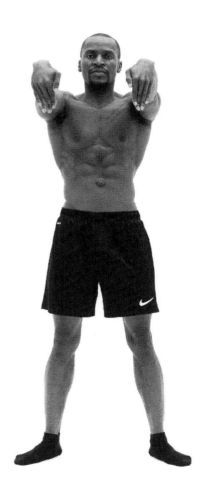 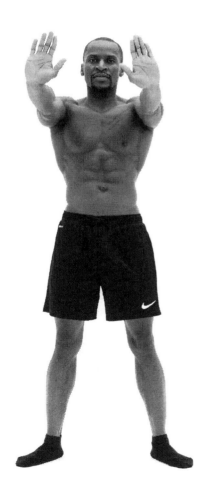

SHOULDER ROTATES

This is a simple but effective warm-up for the rotator cuff and shoulders.

Perform: 10 seconds in each direction.

1. Stand firm and extend both arms straight out to your sides.

2. Rotate arms forwards for 10 seconds.

3. Stop and do the same in reverse.

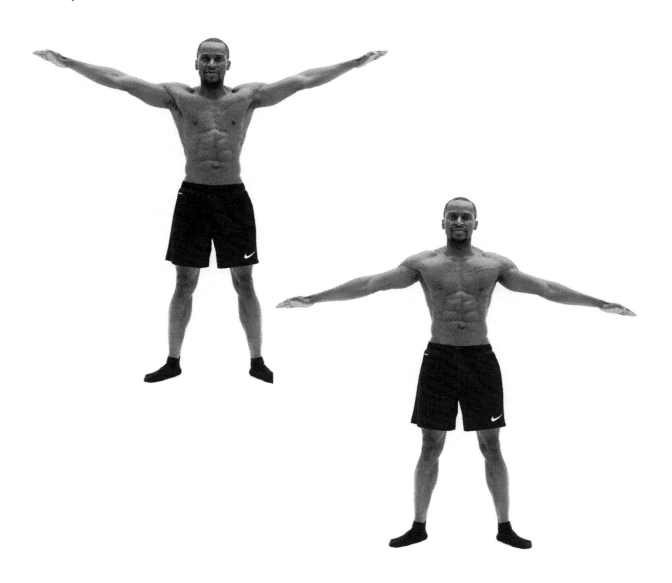

SHOULDER DISLOCATES

Don't panic, the clue isn't actually in the name this time! Your shoulders won't really pop out during this exercise, but they may still be a little uncomfortable at first. Since you will be opening up your shoulders, back, chest and arms here you will probably feel tightness in one or more areas.

Perform: 2 sets of 8 repetitions.

You will need: a long, lightweight bar.

1. Stand up straight, feet shoulder width apart, hands a little wider apart on the bar with an overhand grip (palms down).

2. Lift the bar up directly over your head and in one smooth motion bring it down to rest on your lower back, keeping your elbows locked at all times.

3. Reverse the movement, bringing the bar back to the front of your body to complete one rep.

You may struggle with this at first, so try sliding your hands wider apart along the bar until you find a position that allows you to perform the movement without bending your arms.

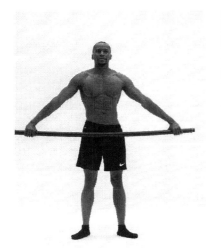 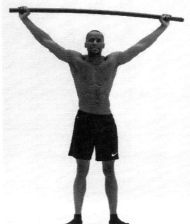 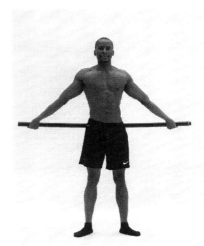

SCAPULA PUSH-UP

The scapula push-up is an excellent way to prepare your upper body for a beating. In particular, this will mobilize the muscles in your upper back and shoulders.

Perform: 8-10 repetitions.

1. Get into push-up position (see push-ups if unsure), placing your knees on the floor if you are just starting out.

2. Keeping your elbows locked and arms straight, let your chest sink towards the floor and squeeze your scapulae together at the same time.

3. With your elbows still locked, reverse this movement, lifting your chest back up and separating your scapula so that your back arches and your spine rises.

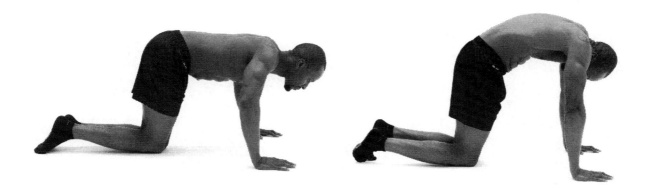

SCAPULA PULL-UP

The clue is in the name again; we'll be working your scapula and upper back here to great effect with an outstanding strengthening mobility exercise.

Perform: 8-10 repetitions.

You will need: a pull-up bar.

1. Grasp the bar overhand and allow yourself to hang with your arms and body totally straight, feet off the floor.

2. Relax, aiming to get your shoulders to touch your ears so your scapulae are elevated.

3. Keeping your arms and elbows locked in position; try to pull your scapulae downward.

4. Hold for 1-2 seconds and then lower back down to the starting position.

The movement involved in this exercise is so subtle that it is best demonstrated with good old-fashioned arrows! You may find this movement very difficult initially, but as with all things your mobility and control will improve over time so stick at it.

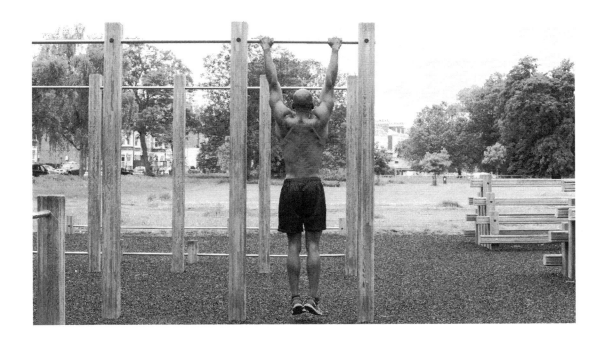

SCAPULA DIP

This motion will fire up your shoulders and give you greater range of movement for 'pushing' exercises such as, well, push-ups!

Perform: 8-10 repetitions.

You will need: parallel bars or dip station.

1. Grab the bars and lock your elbows, lifting your feet up and supporting your body-weight in a neutral position.

2. Keeping your elbows locked and arms straight, sink your body down aiming to get your shoulders to meet your ears (or as close as you can).

3. With your arms still locked straight, push back upwards as high as possible, effectively trying to get your shoulders and ears as far apart as you are able.

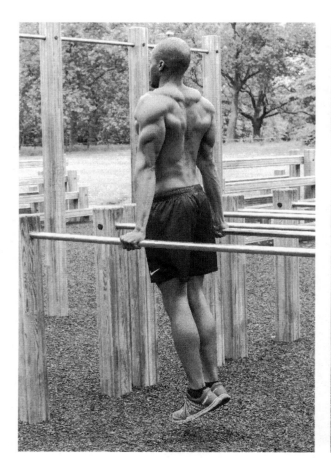
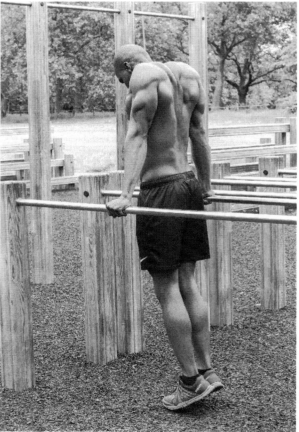

CORE

If you are taking your warm-up seriously then you should have broken a sweat by now. You will be glad to know that core mobility is nice and quick to address! Let's get to it.

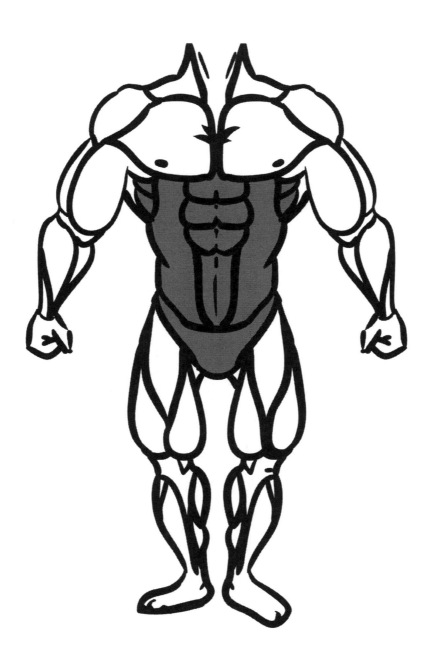

HIP ROTATES

Get your hula on to open up those hip flexors and increase your range of motion.

Perform: 2 sets of 8 repetitions in each direction.

1. Stand upright and place one hand on each hip.

2. Slowly rotate your hips clockwise in a 'hula' movement, aiming to keep your knees and back neutral, focusing the movement in your hips.

3. Repeat the movement counter-clockwise.

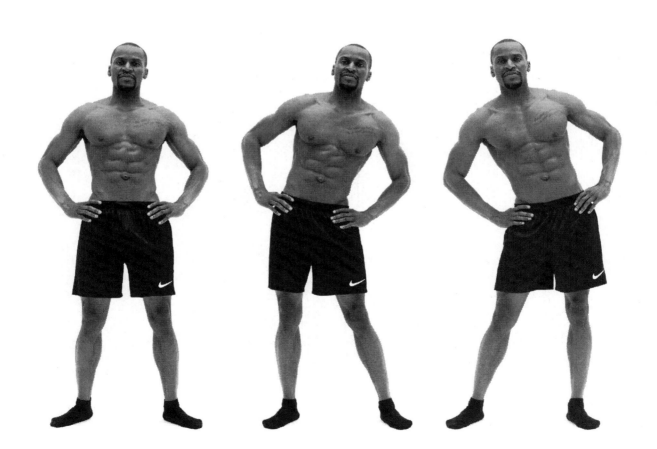

SIDE LEANS

Tight obliques and an inflexible lower spine can greatly inhibit your range of motion, so perform this movement to loosen up these areas.

Perform: 5 repetitions in each direction.

You will need: a long, lightweight bar.

1. Stand upright with your feet just wider than shoulder width apart, grasping the bar over your head.

2. Keeping your arms straight, feet rooted and shoulders in position, lean over to one side to stretch out the other.

3. When you have reached as low as possible, reverse the movement and repeat the exercise on the other side of your body.

Variation: You can perform this exercise without a bar if needs be, simply lean over to one side and grab your leg with the closest hand, bringing the other arm up overhead.

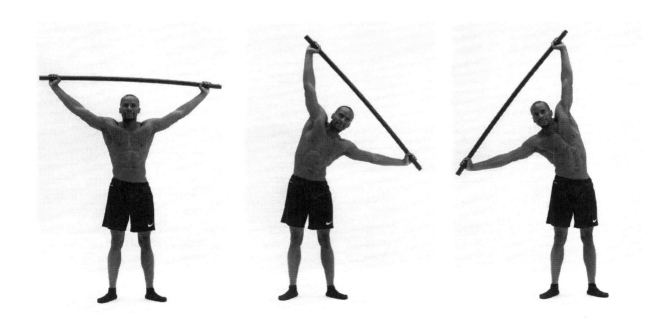

LOWER BODY

Even if you're not training lower body you will still be using it to get around so it's good practice to perform these exercises, too. Check out the following and incorporate them into your routine, or simply practice them on off days.

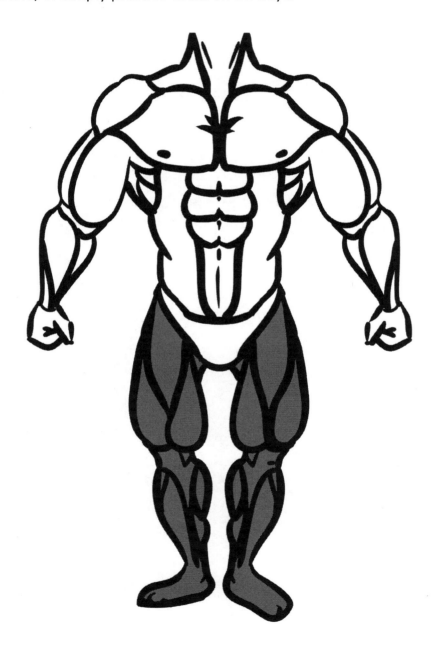

OPEN / CLOSE GATES

This is a staple mobility exercise for elite athletes across a whole range of sports, so it is well worth adding into your routine.

Perform: 8-10 repetitions on each leg.

1. Stand upright and raise one leg upwards, knee bent at 90 degrees.

2. Bring the leg out to the side to open up your hips and groin.

3. Perform the same movement in reverse, first bringing the leg up to the side, then around to the front and back down to the ground.

Variation: You can also perform this exercise on your hands and knees, lifting one knee off the ground, extending it backwards and then bringing it all the way back round the front, and vice versa.

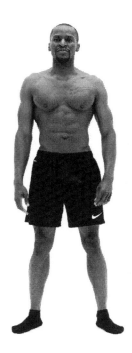 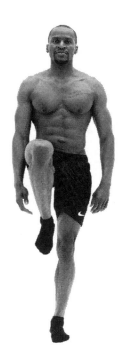 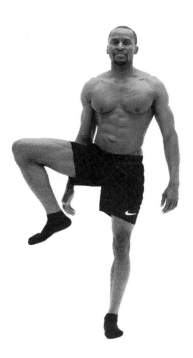

DEEP SQUAT

The squat is an exercise in itself, but we can make it – and almost every other lower body exercise – more effective by practicing the deep squat routinely. Because this one takes a little longer than the others you may prefer to do it on off days or after a heavy lower body session.

Perform: 3-5 minutes or more hold time.

1. Stand with your feet just beyond shoulder width apart, toes pointing out slightly at a comfortable, neutral angle.

2. Bend your knees and lower down into a squat position, ensuring you keep your lower back straight and push your hips back while doing so.

3. Once in position, clasp your hands together and rest your elbows just inside your knees, creating leverage to push your legs outward slightly.

4. Hold for 5 minutes, or as long as you can comfortably.

Variation: If you struggle to maintain your balance at first, place your legs either side of a sturdy pole or fixture and hold onto that to ensure you maintain the proper form.

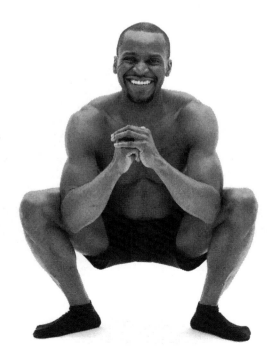

MOUNTAIN CLIMBERS

This is a fantastic, and dynamic, movement to warm up your body and get the blood flowing. Keep your reps unbroken and really lean into the movement to achieve the maximum benefit and increase your hip mobility.

Perform: 8 reps.

1. Assume the push-up position with your arms completely locked out, bringing your left leg forward and placing your foot beside your left hand.

2. Push both feet off the ground and quickly switch them. Now your right foot should be forward and your left out back. This counts as one rep.

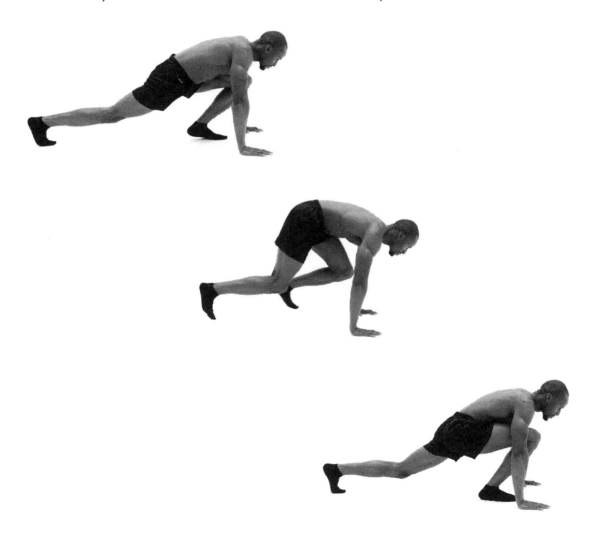

FROG HOPS

This is another excellent exercise to improve your hip mobility, and prepare your body for any exercise involving the lower body.

Perform: 8 reps.

1. Assume the push-up position with arms fully locked out.

2. Leave your hands in place, and jump forward with your feet, landing with them just outside your hands.

3. Reverse the movement and return to the start to complete one rep.

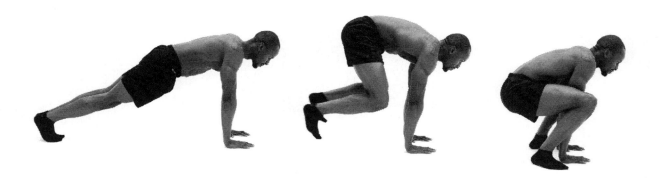

Flexibility & Stretching

Flexibility is a key component of a wide range of motion and, therefore, strength. Static stretching is the act of holding certain positions, generally for 15-30 seconds, in order to increase flexibility and minimize risk of injury.

You should be stretching after your workout or, if you are feeling tight in certain areas pre-workout, stretch them out then. Check out the following examples to target each area of your body. You can also do this on off days to accelerate your progress.

Remember: If you still feel tight in certain areas after stretching, throw in another set.

Tip: Relax during stretching. This might sound counter-productive but it is relaxing the muscles that allow them to stretch further. Try letting out a long, deep breath as you stretch a muscle and feel how much further it takes you!

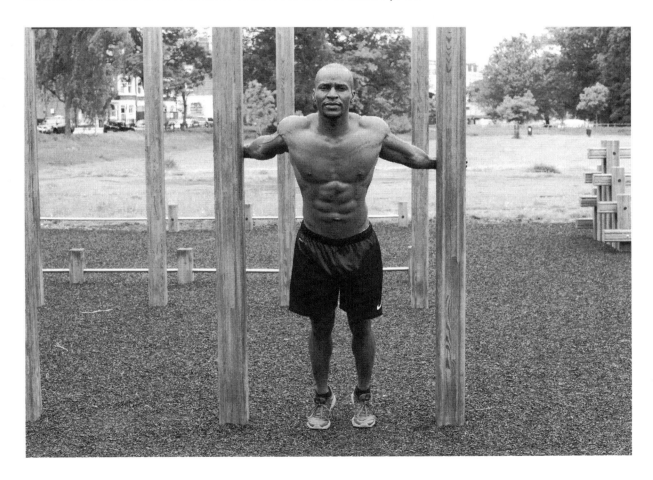

UPPER BODY

The upper body takes a beating during calisthenics training, so ensuring you are fully prepped is key. By improving your flexibility you will also get more out of your workouts, therefore enjoying greater results. We'll start from the top and work our way down.

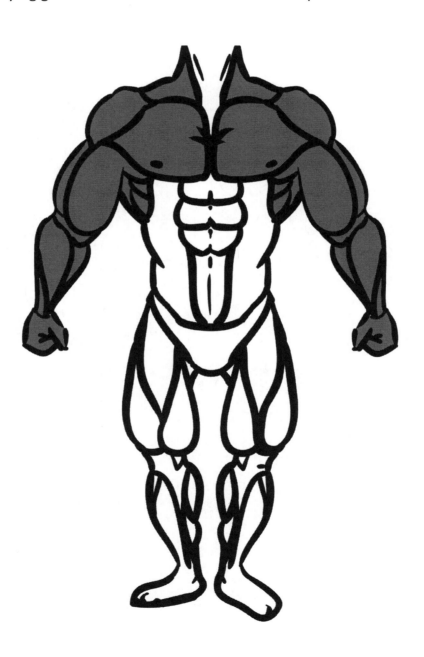

WRISTS & FOREARMS

Great as preparation for handstands as well as all-round strength, get to know both these variations to strengthen your wrists.

Perform: 30 second hold time.

1. Get on your knees and place your palms flat, fingers facing forward, just in front of your knees.

2. Lock your arms and slowly lean forwards as far as you can without raising your palms, and hold for the allotted time.

3. Return to start position and repeat the exercise, this time with your fingers facing towards you and leaning backwards instead of forwards.

Variation: If you find this too difficult then use a wall to perform a similar stretch.

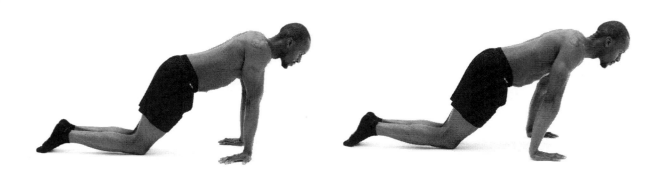

CHEST & SHOULDERS

This stretch is essential in opening up two of the largest muscle groups in your upper body. Find somewhere comfortable and relax into it.

Perform: 30 second hold time.

1. Get onto your hands and knees, then stretch your arms out in front of you.

2. With your hands and knees rooted to the spot, bring your chest down towards the ground, exhaling as you go.

3. When your chest and shoulders are as low as possible, hold this pose for the allotted time. Remember to relax.

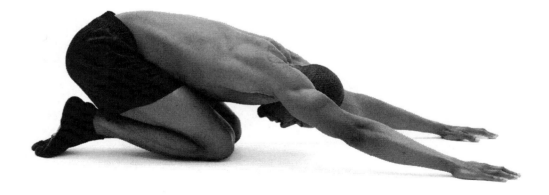

CHEST II

Your chest bears the brunt of almost every upper body exercise in calisthenics, so keep it properly conditioned with this simple stretch.

Perform: 30 second hold time.

You will need: upright parallel bars or doorframe.

1. Stand between the bars or doorframe and stretch your arms out to the sides, placing your palms flat on the surface.

2. Ensuring your arms stay straight, lean forward and stretch out your chest, holding for the allotted time.

Variations:

• If you don't have parallel bars use a single bar to stretch one side at a time. Instead of leaning forward, simply turn your body away from your affixed hand to stretch out one side of your chest then repeat on the other.

• You can also perform this exercise on a flat surface, rooting one hand against it and rotating away from that hand.

• Place a medicine ball or other platform on the floor and kneel beside it. Place one arm up on the platform, and then lower your body down to stretch out that side of your chest.

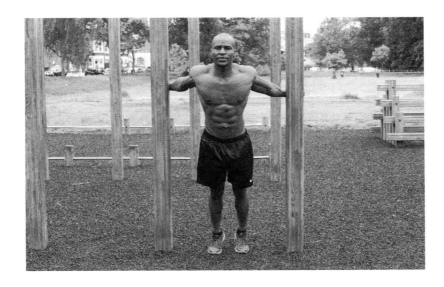

UPPER BACK

This is another area that will take a beating as you condition your body, so get into the habit of stretching it out.

Perform: 30 second hold time.

You will need: a study bar or fixture.

1. Grab a straight bar or other immovable fixture with one hand.

2. Keeping your arm locked, slowly lean back to stretch out your lattisumus dorsi (lat) on that side.

3. Bring your free arm around in front of your body to stretch further and hold for the allotted time. Repeat on the other side for an effective back stretch.

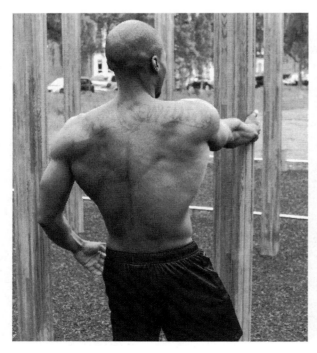 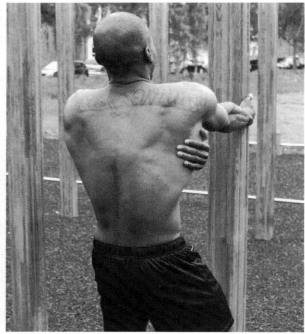

CORE

Everyone covets a chiseled core, and combining mobility and flexibility exercises with bodyweight training will help you achieve just that. You'll find this part quick and easy.

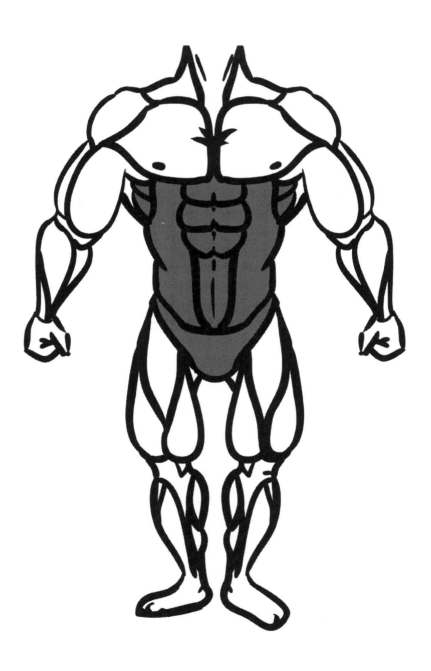

SIDE STRETCH

Prepare your lats, obliques, and lower back for movement with this standing side stretch, the same movement covered in mobility previously. As with all stretches, you don't want to be flexing, or straining against the movement. Instead, let your muscles relax and fall into the stretch for maximum benefit.

Perform: 15 second holds per side.

You will need: a long, lightweight bar.

1. Stand upright with your feet just wider than shoulder-width apart, grasping the bar over your head.

2. Keeping your arms straight, feet rooted and shoulders in position, lean over to one side to stretch out the other.

3. When you have reached as low as possible, reverse the movement and repeat the exercise on the other side of your body.

Variation: You can perform this exercise without a bar if needs be, simply lean over to one side and grab your leg with the closest hand, bringing the other arm up overhead.

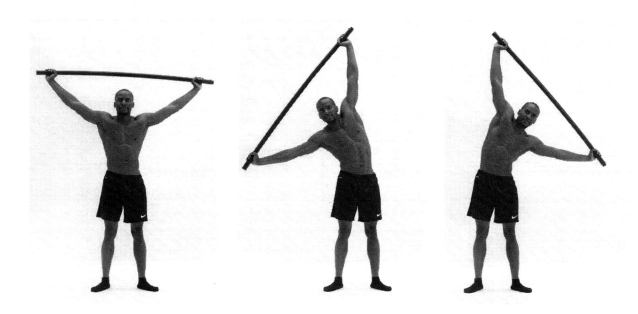

COBRA

If you've ever done yoga you'll know this one as the 'cobra' already. For everyone else, here it is, ideal for opening up your lower back and hips.

Perform: 15-30 second hold time.

1. Lie on your stomach and place your palms flat on the floor, similar to a standard push-up position, fingers facing forward, about shoulder-width apart.

2. With your hips rooted to the ground, raise your head and look upwards, allowing your spine to arch and hold for allotted time.

Variation: If you find this tough to hold, practice raising up onto your forearms and holding the stretch there first.

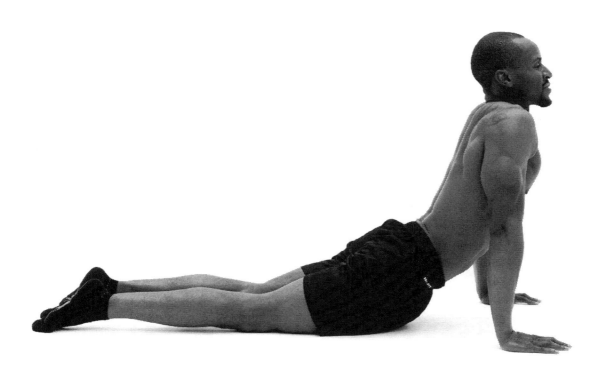

CAT

Another yoga stretch named 'cat', essentially designed to stretch the opposite way to cobra, opening up your back nicely.

Perform: 15-30 second hold time.

1. Get on your hands and knees, palms flat directly underneath your shoulders, fingers facing forward.

2. Drop your head and arch your back as if trying to look at your naval, and hold for the allotted amount of time.

Variation: To turn this into a mobility exercises, get into position and then transition to a downwardly arched back, raising your head up. Moving between the two in a fluid motion is a great way to warm up.

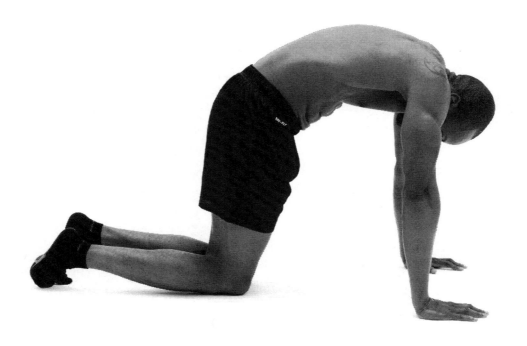

LOWER BODY

Last but by no means least is lower body flexibility. Not only will this help you achieve your dream body, it will also prove useful in everyday life, especially as the years go by. Don't let tight hamstrings, hip flexors or other problem areas hold you back. Let's go!

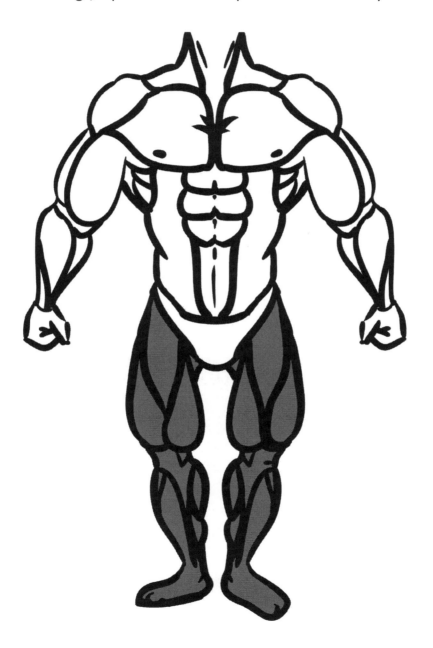

CALVES

Essential for strength and stability, you must ensure your calves are flexible enough to cope with the demands of calisthenics. And, of course, for showing off at barbeques!

Perform: 30 seconds hold time for each leg.

1. Get into push-up position.

2. Take one foot and rest the top of it on the heel of the other.

3. Slowly push the heel of the standing foot down as far as possible and hold for allotted time.

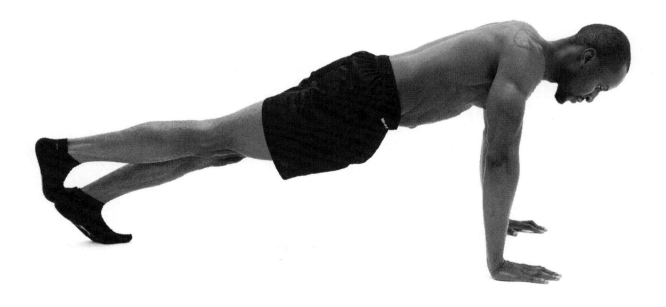

HAMSTRINGS

Most people have tight hamstrings, which can severely inhibit your range of lower body motion. Loosen them up like so:

Perform: 30 second hold time on each leg.

1. Sit down with both legs stretched out in front of you, toes pointing upwards.

2. Bring one foot towards you so the sole is against the inner thigh of the other leg.

3. Keeping your back straight, lean forwards towards the toes of your outstretched leg and hold for allotted time.

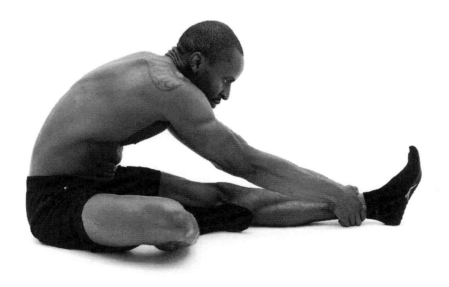

GROIN

Opening up your groin will also open up your hips. You are probably beginning to see how everything is linked together now, so you should never neglect one area in favor of another.

Perform: 30 second hold time.

1. Sit down and bring the soles of your feet together.

2. Keeping your back straight, pull your feet towards your body as close as possible.

3. Try to move your knees outwards to touch the floor. If you cannot do this with leg power alone, use your elbows or hands for a little assistance.

4. Hold for allotted time. You may find one side tighter than the other here, but don't worry, it will even out over time.

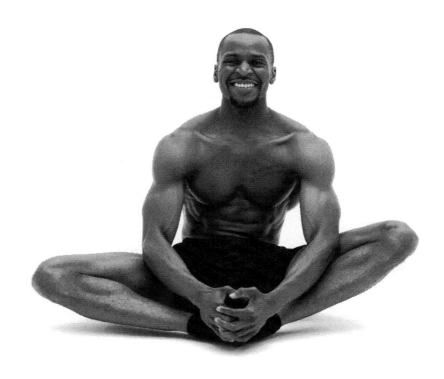

GLUTES

This is a hugely powerful part of your body, driving some of the most important motions required for lower body activities, which is why professional athletes and sports stars often have backsides like Beyoncé.

Perform: 30 second hold time on each side.

1. Lay on your back.

2. Bend the knee of one leg and bring it towards you, grasping the leg underneath your hamstring area with both hands.

3. Bring the other leg up and over so the ankle is resting just above the knee of the leg you are holding.

4. Pull the leg you are holding towards you to create a stretch in the opposite side and hold for allotted time.

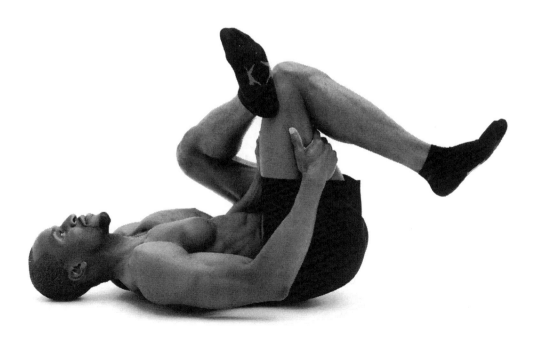

HIP FLEXOR

Your hip flexors work in harmony with your glutes so you can't stretch one without the other. Check this out:

Perform: 30 second hold time on each side

1. Stand upright, then place one foot forward.

2. Bend the knee of your front foot and, keeping your body straight and rear foot on the spot, lean forward.

3. When you feel a stretch in the top of your back leg, hold for allotted time.

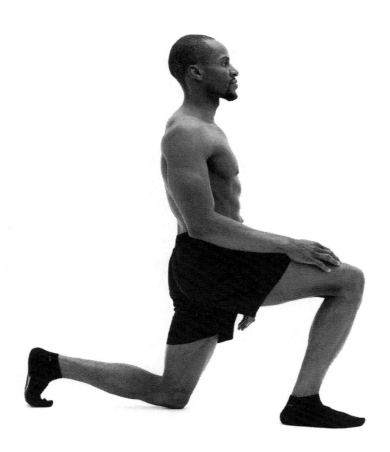

Hips II

Here, we'll focus on your hips, groin, and hammies, areas that are chronically tight in many people.

Perform: 30 second hold.

1. Start at a comfortable sitting position on the floor, and then spread your legs outward as far as you can.

2. Slowly lean forward as far as possible into the space between your legs, and hold for allotted time.

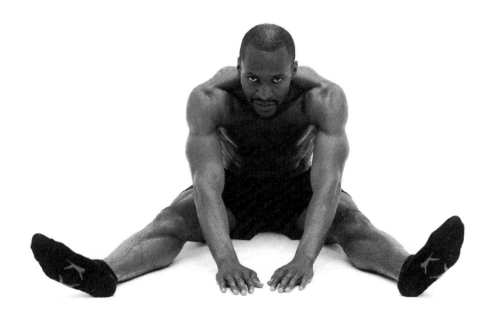

QUADRICEPS

Another massive muscle group vitally important to both calisthenics and day-to-day life are your quads. Keep them happy with this simple stretch:

Perform: 30 second hold time.

1. Lie down flat on your stomach.

2. Bend one knee and bring the foot towards your glutes.

3. Grasp the foot with your hand and pull it towards your glutes, then hold for allotted time.

That covers the essential stretching for major muscle groups. Remember to stretch after each workout to aid recovery and increase range of motion and, subsequently, strength.

Listen to your body and seek advice from a specialist if you are unsure about anything. You should be using this advice as a general guideline to help build your own stretching routine rather than sticking to it exactly as it's written above.

For a comprehensive guide on building superhuman strength through flexibility, pick up our companion book on Amazon. Just search 'Pure Calisthenics Flexibility'.

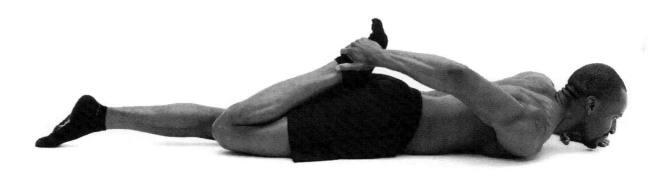

"Take care of your body. It's the only place you have to live."

Jim Rohn

5. EXERCISES

It's time to get into the good stuff! If you commit to mastering the following exercises and don't throw in the towel when the going gets tough then you WILL experience mind-blowing results.

Disclaimer: This bodyweight training guide has been designed to help you learn the art of calisthenics progressively. Each exercise will start off with the simplest variation, becoming more difficult as you work through the book.

Since we cannot be there to train you in person, we have provided HD photographs and detailed tutorials. We cannot be held accountable for any misuse of instructions or injuries that occur as a result. It is down to you to be smart and attempt only what you are ready for.

Where possible, always use a spotter or personal trainer to ensure you are using the correct form for each exercise. There is no glory or value in squeezing out more sets or reps than someone else if you aren't performing the exercises properly.

Remember: This is a resource created to teach bodyweight exercises, NOT a training program. We cannot suggest an exact amount of sets and reps for you without knowing your level of ability, so the numbers given in this guide are just a suggestion.

If you want to get started with a proper training routine you will find a link at the back of this book to our free companion program. As always, for a more personal approach, hook up with a calisthenics trainer to create a bespoke program.

All that is left to do at this stage is make sure you are sufficiently warmed up before jumping into any of the following exercises. If you skipped the section on warm-up and preparation, do yourself a favor and go back a few steps. It might just be the difference between make or break.

So, you're clued up, you're warmed up, and you're raring to go. Just what kind of crazy exercises are we going to use to achieve SUPERHUMAN form?

Well, the most astonishing thing is, it all starts with the humble push-up.

Let's do this!

UPPER BODY

Ready to build a bulging upper body? It all begins here, so read on and always master the fundamentals before advancing. Don't forget your mobility and flexibility work!

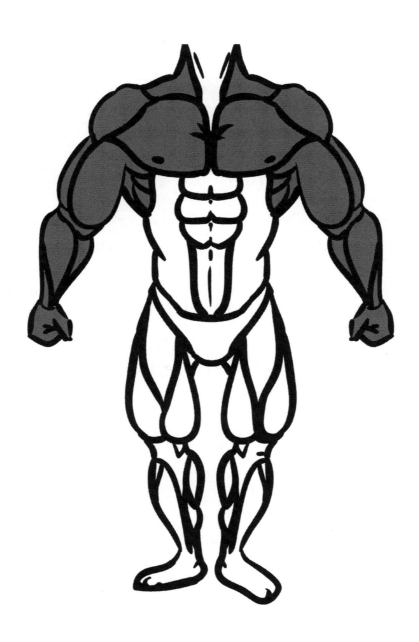

PUSH-UPS

Push-ups are part of our 'essential 12' bodyweight exercises. In fact, they are the very first thing we recommend mastering, since most people already have a grasp on them at some level. Remember not to race ahead to more challenging exercises before you have nailed the basics. If you are attempting things beyond your capabilities your form will suffer and you will do more harm to your body than good. With that said, let's go!

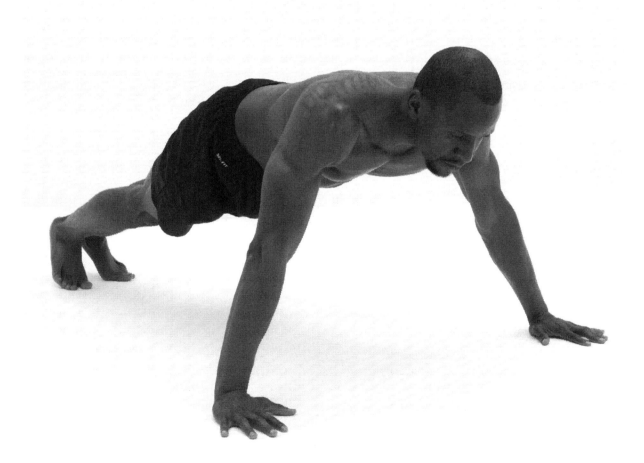

STANDARD PUSH-UP

This is one of the pillars of calisthenics, and it is essential learn it with the proper form. Check it out here and see if you can complete the allocated sets and reps.

Perform: 3-4 sets of 8-12 repetitions (reps).

1. Place your palms flat on the floor, shoulder width apart.

2. Push up onto your hands and toes, keeping your feet close together and your legs, hips and shoulders in a straight line.

3. With your chin slightly raised so you are not staring straight at the ground, bend your elbows and lower yourself to the ground.

4. Stop when your chest makes contact with the ground but do not lie down or drop to the floor completely. Remember to keep your body in a straight line and do not let your stomach touch the ground – you should be engaging your core muscles to prevent this.

5. Push yourself back up hard, ensuring your body remains locked in a straight line. You have now completed one repetition!

Variations:

If you are new to push-ups or exercise in general then there is no shame in struggling to complete this movement. Instead of battling through with bad form, try the platform or box push-ups for an easier alternative as shown next. Once you have mastered 3 sets of 10 reps with the proper form, go back and try the standard push-up again.

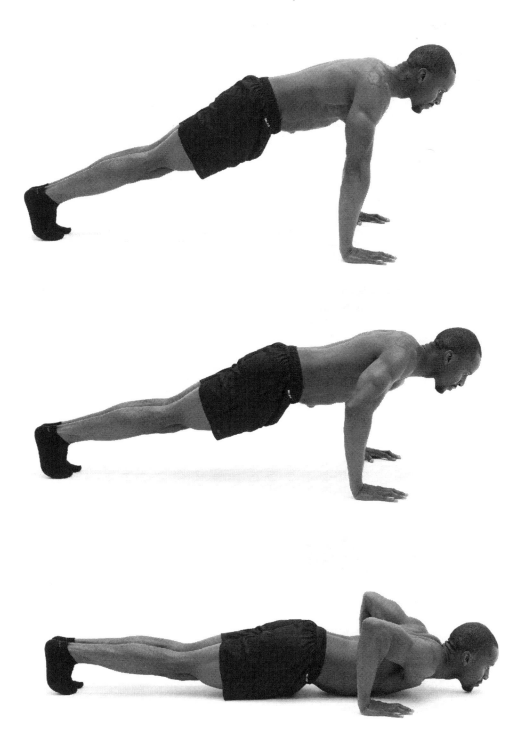

Box Push-Up

Not to be confused with the platform push-up (next), this is the easiest version of the movement.

Perform: 3-4 sets of 8-12 repetitions (reps).

1. Get onto your hands and knees, keeping your feet close together.

2. Bend your elbows and lower yourself to the ground.

3. Stop when your head gets close to the ground. You can increase the angle and make things more difficult by bringing your knees back further.

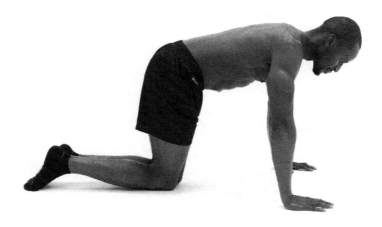

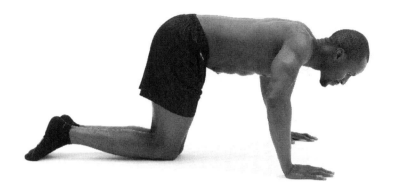

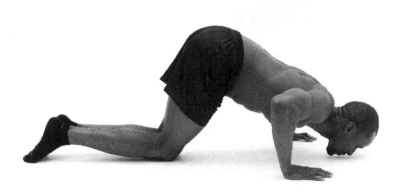

PLATFORM INCLINE PUSH-UP

You can use any raised surface to perform this version. It's perfect if you are struggling with form or simply want to switch up your technique.

Perform: 3-4 sets of 8-12 repetitions (reps).

You will need: a sturdy platform.

1. Place your feet on the floor and your hands on a sturdy platform.

2. Bend your elbows and lower yourself towards the platform.

3. Stop when your chest reaches the platform. Note that the higher it is, the easier this variation will be.

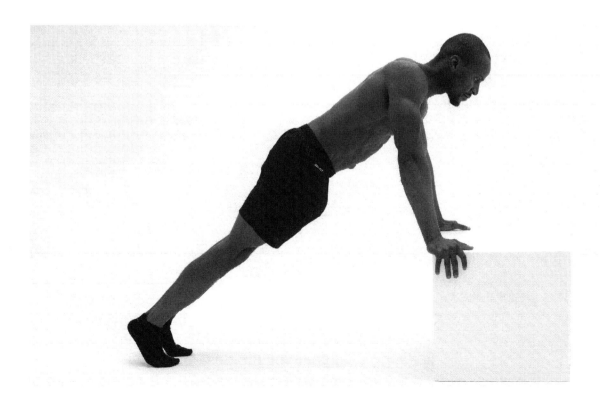

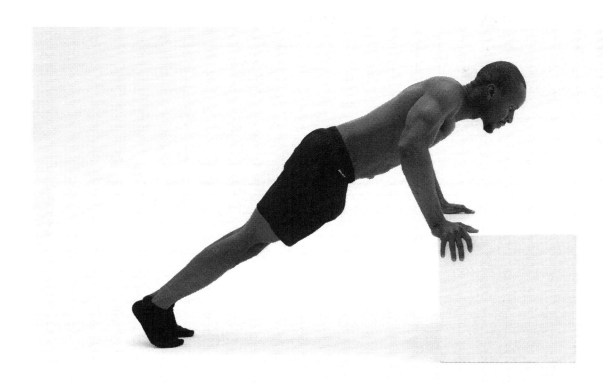

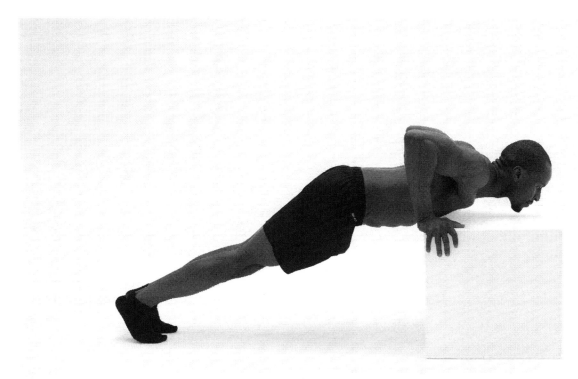

PLATFORM DECLINE PUSH-UP

Swap your hands and feet around on the platform to increase the challenge and send your chest and shoulders into overdrive!

Perform: 3-4 sets of 8-12 repetitions (reps).

You will need: a sturdy platform.

1. Place your feet on the platform and your hands on the floor in front of you.

2. Bend your elbows and lower yourself towards the platform.

3. Stop when your chest reaches the platform. Note that the higher the platform is, the more difficult this will become.

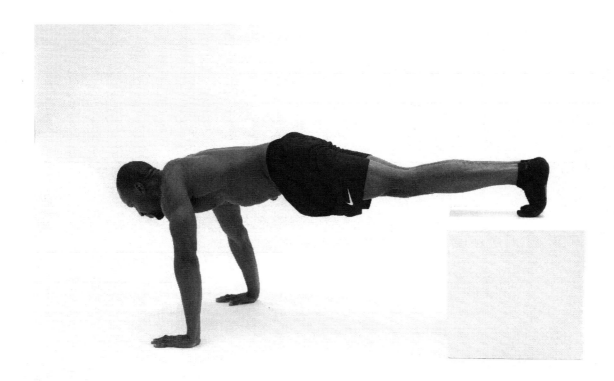

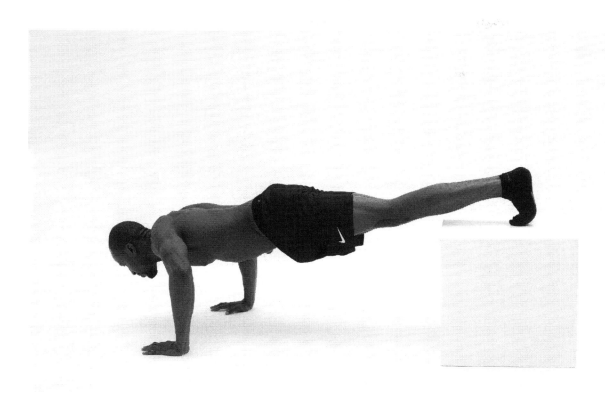

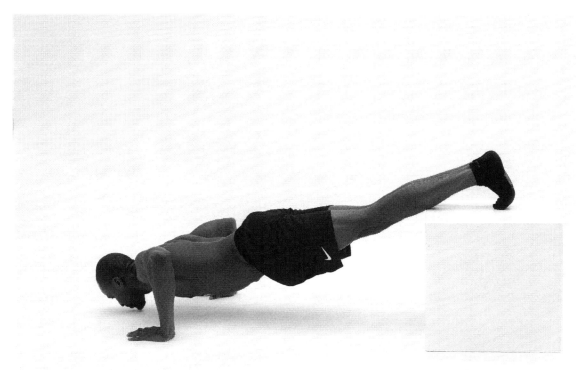

CLOSE GRIP PUSH-UP

Once you have mastered the basic grip you can begin to explore new hand positions.

Perform: 3-4 sets of 8-12 reps.

1. Get into the push-up position, and then bring your hands together to form a diamond shape between your fingers.

2. Bend your elbows and, keeping your elbows tucked in close to your sides, lower your chest to the ground ensuring your body remains straight as always.

3. Once your chest has touched the ground, push yourself back up.

Variations:

• This may be uncomfortable or even painful at first, so if you struggle you can try an easier version. Simply move your hands further apart until you are able to perform 3 sets of 10 reps. Move your hands closer together to increase the difficulty over time.

• Another alternative is to use a raised platform, or support yourself on your knees as shown previously.

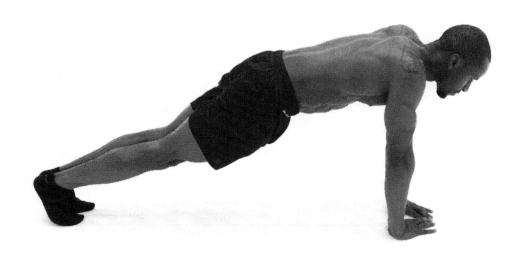

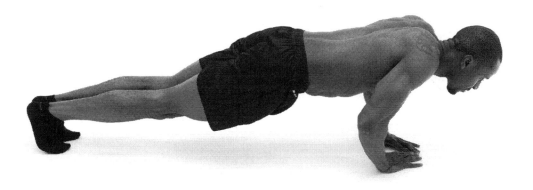

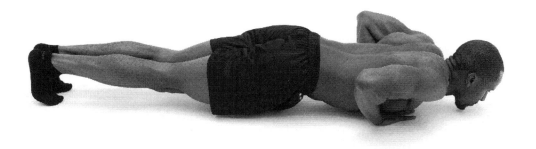

WIDE GRIP PUSH-UP

This is another variation on the standard push-up. Combining this with the previous two gives you a great basis for a ripped chest arm bulging arms!

Perform: 3-4 sets of 8-12 reps.

1. Get into standard push-up position, then place your hands as wide apart as possible ensuring your chest stays off the ground and your shoulders, hips and legs remain in a straight line.

2. Bend your elbows and lower your chest to the ground.

3. Push yourself back up to the starting position to complete a rep.

Variations:

• If you find this too difficult, try moving your hands inwards a little until you reach a point where you can complete the allotted reps. Over time you will be able to progress to a wider grip.

• The variations shown in the standard push-up are also an option here.

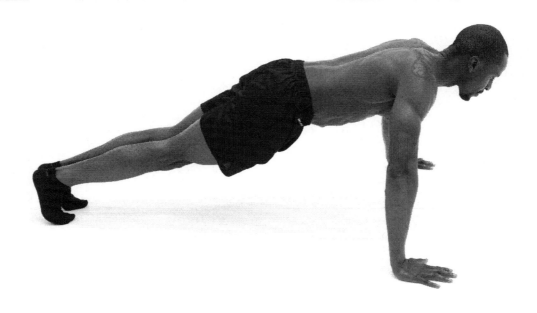

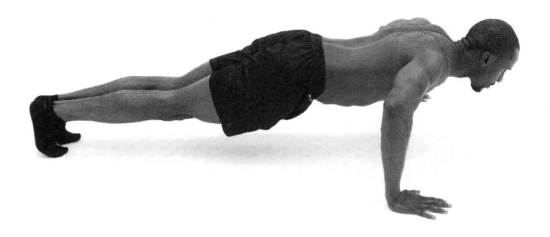

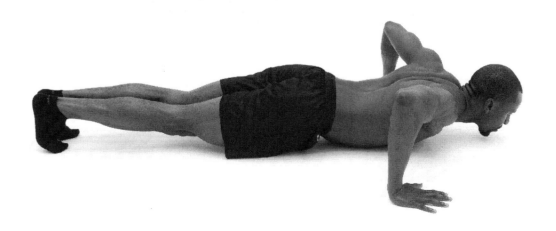

FINGERTIP PUSH-UP

For all the rock climbers out there, this exercise has the added benefit of strengthening your fingers and hands for those extra crimpy routes! Even if you're not into climbing, building strength in your hands is a pivotal step as you move forward to many of the more advanced exercises that require a firm grip.

Perform: 3-4 sets of 6-10 reps.

1. Assume the standard push-up position, supporting yourself using only your fingers and not your whole hand.

2. Now bend your elbows and lower yourself to the ground. As always, chest to deck!

3. Push yourself back to your starting position like a normal push-up to complete one rep. Remember to keep the momentum going!

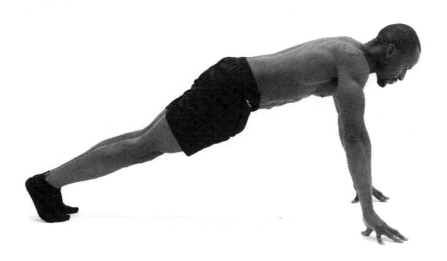

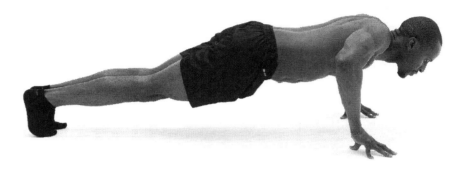

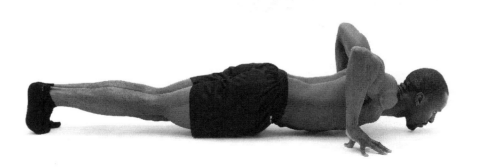

BEGINNER PLANCHE PUSH-UP

This exercise will strengthen the main muscle groups associated with the planche. More specifically, we're focusing on your triceps, chest, biceps, and core.

Perform: 3-4 sets of 3-5 reps.

1. Assume the standard push-up position with your elbows and hands directly beneath your shoulders.

2. Now move your body forward, keeping your hands in place, until your shoulders are forward of your hands. Keep your arms locked out during this shift.

3. Now bend your elbows and lower yourself to the ground (chest to deck!). Try to keep your elbows tucked into your body as you complete this motion.

4. Once your chest is as low as it can go with the proper form, return to the starting position to complete one rep.

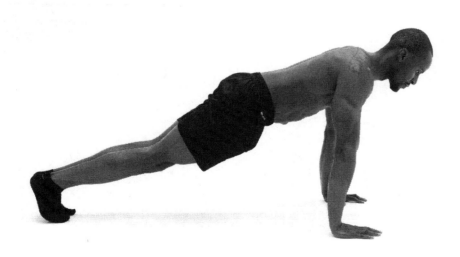

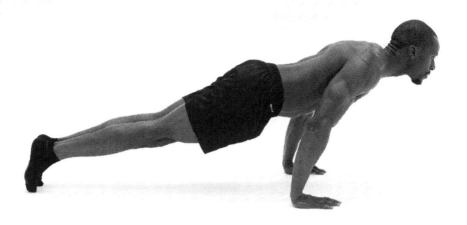

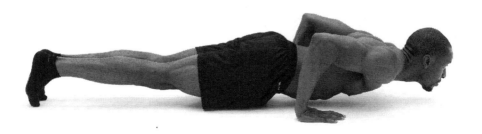

WRIST PUSH-UP

To prepare your wrists for the heavy load-bearing exercises to come, we need to work on strengthening them. To do this, we're going to introduce another variation on the standard push-up, but your wrists will be the main point of support instead of your hands. Remember, this will be a very difficult maneuver to start with, so begin slowly and work your way up as your wrist stability and strength improves.

Perform: 2-3 sets of 3-5 reps.

1. Start on your knees and place your hands on the ground in front of you approximately shoulder width apart. Now flip your hands so your palms are facing upward and your fingers point towards each other (inwards).

2. Once comfortable, raise up onto your wrists and feet slowly, as in the first photo.

3. Now lower yourself to the ground as you would with a standard push-up.

4. Once your chest hits the deck, push back up to starting position to complete a rep.

Variations:

• As always, using a raised platform can make any push-up related exercise simpler.

• You can also leave your knees on the ground while performing this movement if it is too difficult.

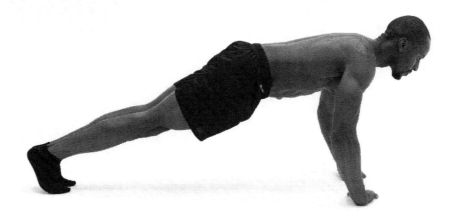

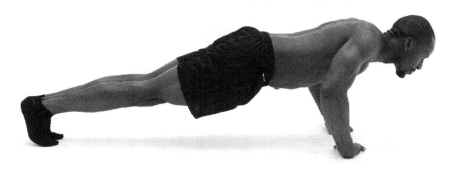

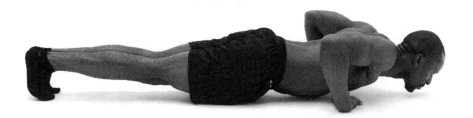

CLAP PUSH-UP

Once you are comfortable with the push-up variations presented so far, it's time to move on to some more explosive movements. The clap push-up will train your core and arms as a standard push up, but will also introduce you to some powerful movements to help you push your muscles hard in a very short amount of time.

Perform: 3-4 sets 6-10 reps.

1. Assume the standard push-up position, with your hands beneath your shoulders and your arms fully locked out.

2. As usual, chest to the ground!

3. When your chest touches the ground, fire your arms as hard as you can to explode upward as fast as possible.

4. As you come up, lift your hands up and clap, then quickly return them to their place on the floor.

5. Bend your arms as you come down to help lessen the jolt of landing, and go straight into your next rep.

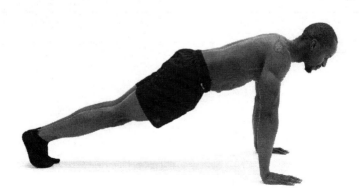

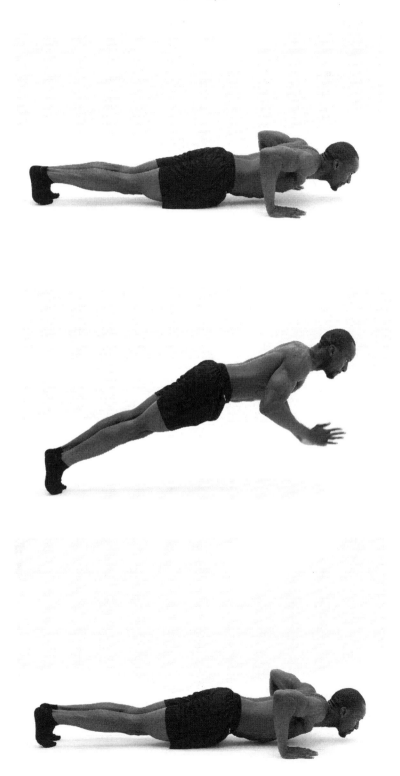

BACK CLAP PUSH-UP

When you can easily complete the clap push-up exercise, it's time to move to the back clap push-up! This will provide an added challenge to the explosiveness of your push-up, and continue to build your upper body strength.

Perform: 3-4 sets 5-8 reps.

1. Assume the standard push-up position, with your hands beneath your shoulders and your arms completely locked out.

2. You know what to do by now. Get low!

3. As before, explode your arms and push as hard as you can against the ground. As your arms are coming up, push off the ground.

4. Throw your hands behind your back and clap once. Whip them back to their starting position and catch yourself as you come back down.

5. Bend your elbows to absorb the shock and drop straight into your next rep.

It's a good idea to do this on a grippy surface, otherwise you might slip when you launch upwards.

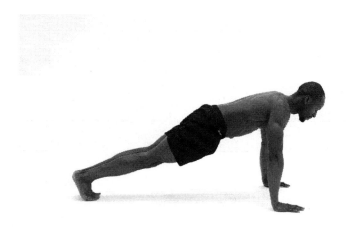

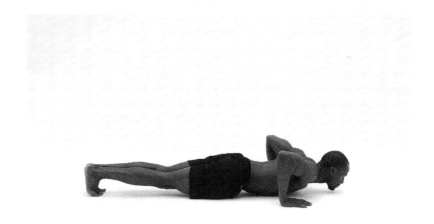

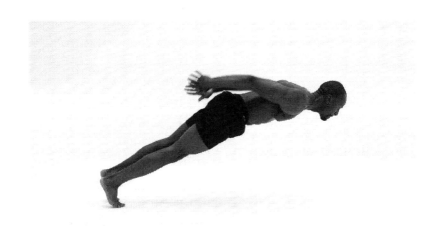

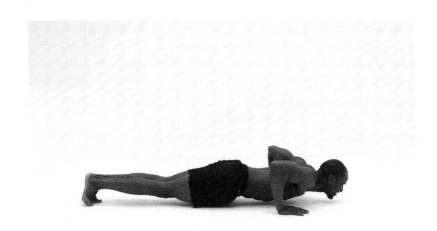

DOUBLE CLAP PUSH-UP

As your strength, stability, and quickness improve with the clap and back clap push-ups, you can progress to the point of combining the two. This movement takes a great deal of swiftness as well as strength, and will without a doubt be an excellent workout. Be careful not to attempt this too soon as you may land on your face!

Perform: 2-3 sets 5-8 reps.

1. Assume the standard push-up position; hands under the shoulders and arms locked out.

2. Chest to deck! Same as any other push-up thus far.

3. Push off the ground with everything you've got. Imagine trying to push yourself all the way to standing.

4. Just as your hands are leaving the ground, perform a quick clap in front of your chest.

5. The instant you have finished this clap, swing your hands behind your back and knock out a second clap.

6. As soon as you've completed this second clap, bring your hands back to their start points and catch your fall. Allow your elbows to bend slightly to absorb the impact, and follow on into your second rep.

NB: Follow the photos left to right, top to bottom.

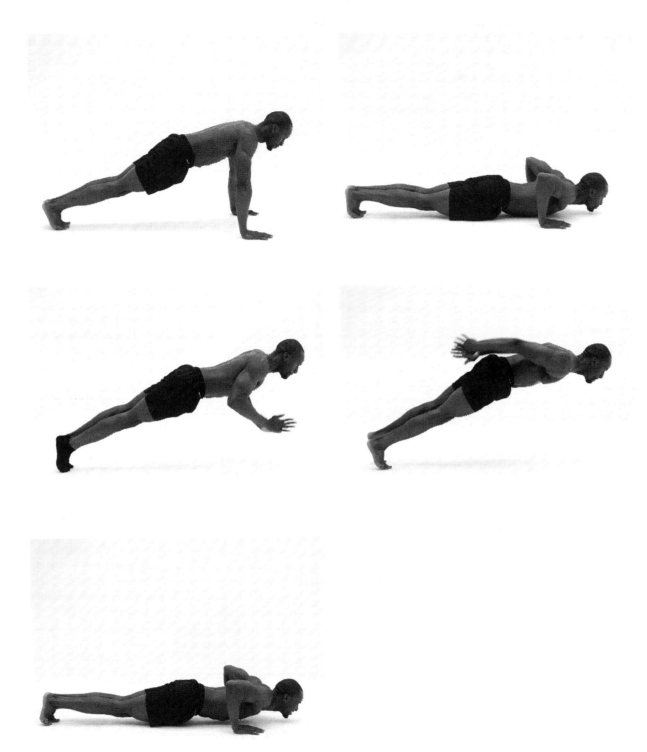

TRIPLE CLAP PUSH-UP

This one is for real beasts only! Once you've nailed the double-clap push-up presented previously, try adding another. Once again this movement will test your strength and speed so we recommend taking care when first starting, and perhaps using a mat to cushion your falls.

Perform: 2-3 sets 2-4 reps.

1. Assume the standard push-up position; hands under the shoulders and arms locked out.

2. Bring your chest on down to the ground.

3. Push off the floor with all your might.

4. Just as your hands are leaving the ground, perform a quick clap in front of your chest.

5. The instant you have finished this clap, swing your hands behind your back to knock out a second clap.

6. The second you finish this second clap, whip your hands back in front and complete the third clap in front of your chest.

7. As soon as you've completed this third clap, bring your hands back to their start points and catch your fall. Allow your elbows to bend slightly to absorb the impact, and go straight into your second rep.

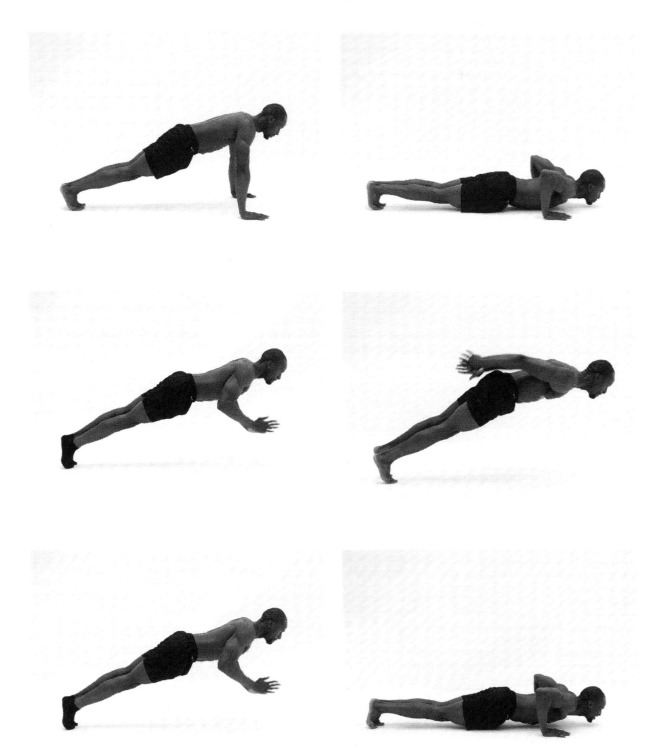

SPIDER-MAN PUSH-UP

Named after the red and blue man in the strange spandex outfit, this is one exercise you will probably be gawked at for doing in public, but it's brilliantly effective nonetheless!

Perform: 2-3 set of 6-10 reps.

1. Assume standard push-up position.

2. Lower your chest to the ground, and at the same time bring your knee up towards the elbow on the same side.

3. Repeat on the other side.

Warning: does not work on the side of tall buildings!

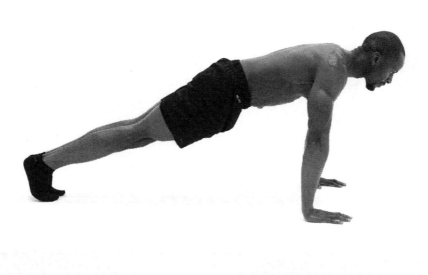

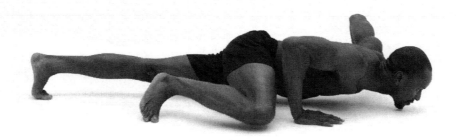

SPIDER PUSH-UP

Not to be confused with the previous exercise, this is a very different movement that will test your fingers, wrists, arms and chest to the extreme.

Perform: 2-3 set of 6-10 reps.

1. Lay on the ground with your arms out at ninety degrees to your body and your palms on the ground. Keep a slight bend in your elbows at this stage.

2. Now press just your fingertips into the ground, tighten your core, and raise yourself until your arms completely locked out. Only your fingers and toes should touch the ground!

3. Lower yourself down to the starting position, completing the rep.

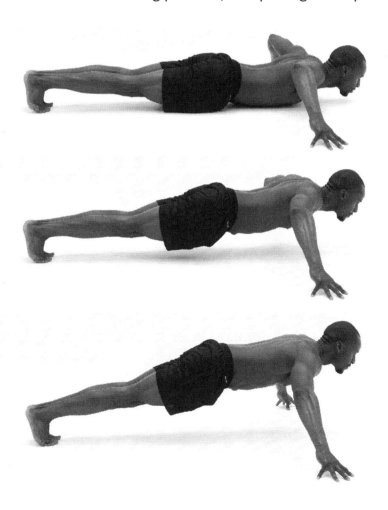

SUPERMAN PUSH-UP

This will develop the strength of your shoulders, triceps, biceps and chest, along with your overall control and balance. Furthermore, this exercise shifts the push-up from a slow and steady movement to something much more dynamic and explosive.

Perform: 2-3 sets of 3-6 reps.

1. Assume the standard push-up position. Hands flat on the floor, arms shoulder width apart, body fully extended with toes on the floor, and arms fully locked out.

2. Slowly lower yourself as you would for a standard push-up, until your chest touches the floor.

3. Now explode upwards as quickly and powerfully as you can. Imagine trying to push so hard that you catapult yourself into a standing position, similar to the clap push-ups.

4. As soon as your hands are about to lift off the floor, shoot your arms in front of you as if you're flying like Superman.

5. Once your arms are completely extended in front of you, bring them back in to catch yourself as you come back down.

6. Allow your arms to bend as you land and go straight into the next rep.

Remember, this exercise is all about explosiveness. Practicing this little and often will enhance your ability to find a rhythm and complete several unbroken reps in one set.

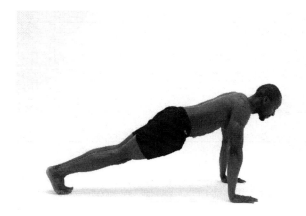
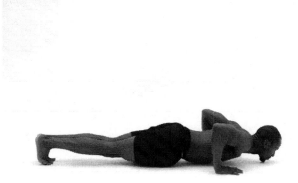

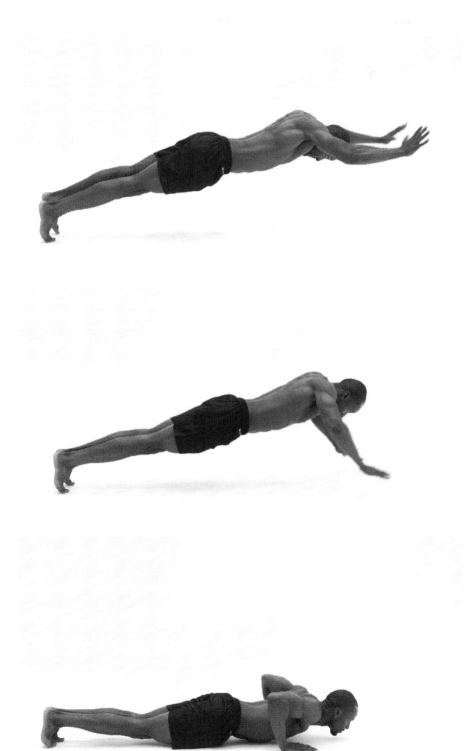

ARCHER PUSH-UP

You will find this type of push-up very reminiscent of the one-arm push-up, but in this case we will be using the unengaged arm for stability and control.

Perform: 2-3 sets of 3-5 reps.

1. Assume push-up position, but place your hands more than shoulder width apart for this movement.

2. Bend your right elbow and begin to lower yourself to the ground. You will naturally drift towards your right side, so try to keep the other arm relatively locked out.

3. When your chest contacts the ground, push with your right arm and begin to raise yourself back up. Keep that left arm locked!

4. When you reach your starting position, repeat the movement, but switch which arm you bend.

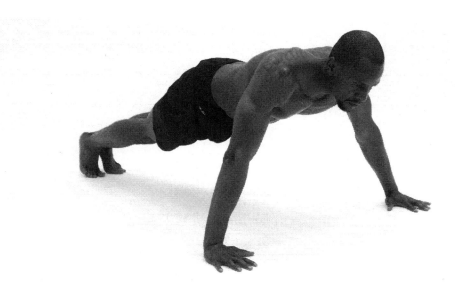

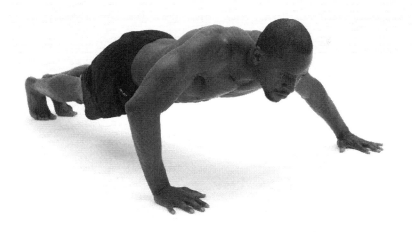

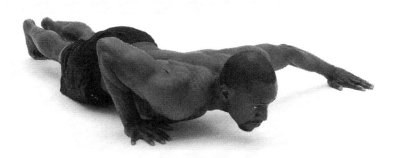

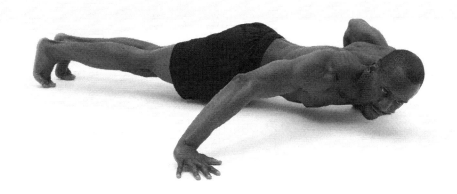

SINGLE-ARM PUSH-UP

The revered one-arm push-up is an extremely challenging movement, and is therefore very beneficial to your fitness. In addition to the obvious workload for your arm and shoulder, this exercise will develop your core and overall stability as you endeavor to maintain your position throughout the movement.

Perform: 2-3 sets of 2-5 reps.

1. Assume the same position you would for the standard push-up, but place only one hand on the floor directly underneath your chest. If you're just beginning, splay your legs out a little to aid in stability.

2. Bend your elbow and lower your body as far as your can, ideally touching your chest to your hand or the ground.

3. Raise yourself back to the starting position. Congratulations, you just rocked one rep!

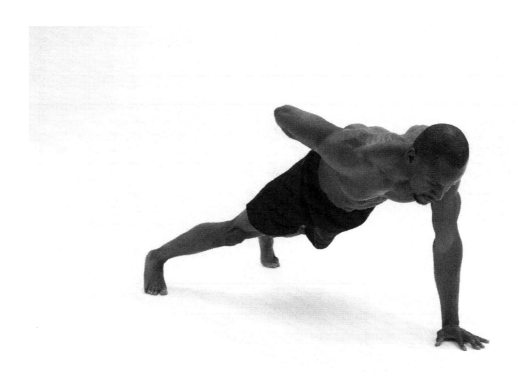

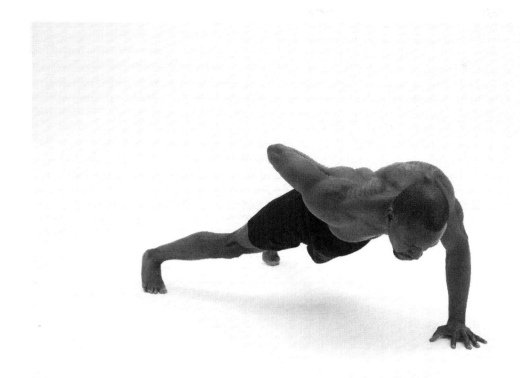

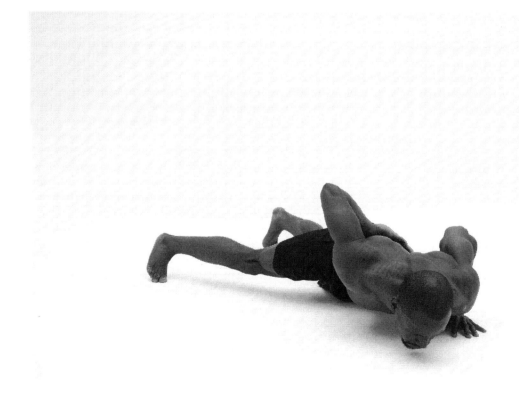

SINGLE-ARM SINGLE-LEG PUSH-UP

When you are able to complete the one-arm push-up comfortably, you can up your game by moving on to this exercise. This will again strain your core and stability as you are eliminating another point of support.

Perform: 2-3 sets of 2-5 reps.

1. Assume the same position outlined for the one-arm push-up, but now lift up the leg on the same side as the arm you're working too.

2. You know what's coming, chest to deck! Lower your body until your chest is touching either your supporting hand or the ground.

3. Now push yourself back up to your starting position to complete a rep.

4. Give yourself a standing ovation because that is one huge achievement!

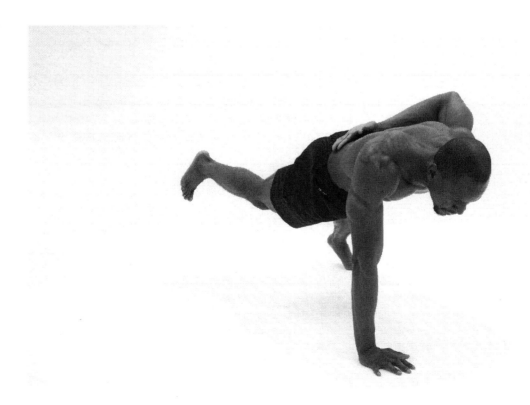

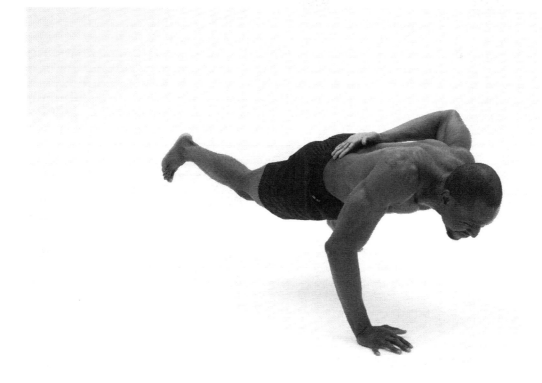

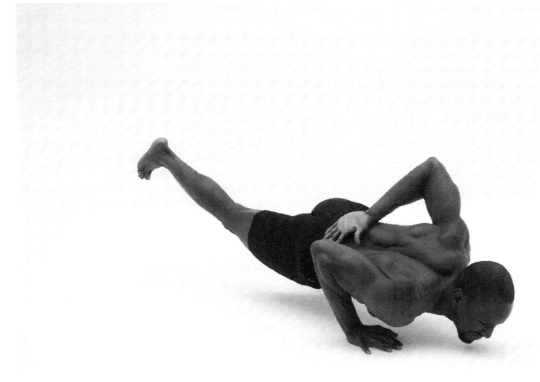

WALL PUSH-UP

This straightforward modification to the standard push-up will up the ante for your core and shoulders, and continue to develop your stability.

Perform: 3-4 sets of 8-12 reps.

You Will Need: a solid wall to brace against.

1. Assume the standard push-up position with your feet nudged up to the base of a wall.

2. Now place your feet on the wall, and bring them up to approximately the same height as your shoulders. Once in position, be sure to maintain a straight back.

3. Begin to lower yourself to the ground by bending at the elbows until you are as low as possible.

4. Once you've gone as low as you can, begin to push yourself up. When you reach start position, you've done 1 rep.

Variation: The above doubles as a decline push-up. For a more traditional push-up, walk your feet down the wall in small increments as you lower down in order to maintain a horizontal position throughout the entire movement.

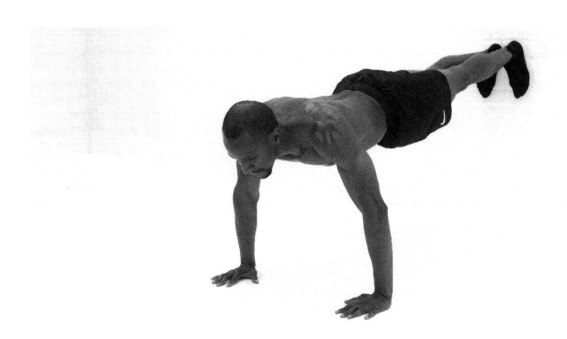

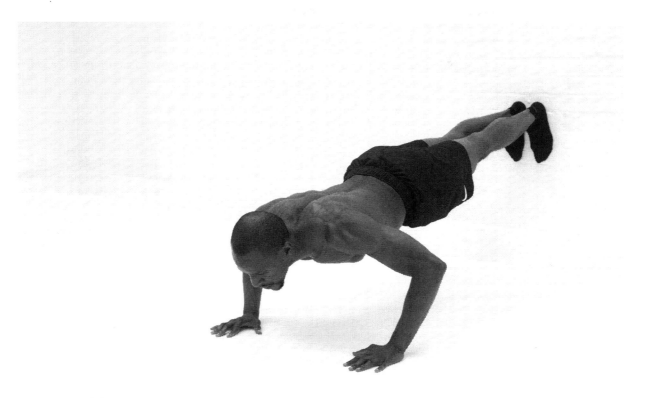

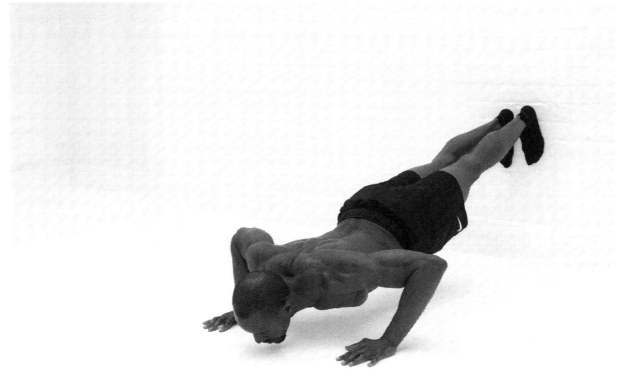

DEEP PUSH-UP

Designed to push you to your limits, this will yield phenomenal results when done with the proper form. Though this is primarily a chest and arm exercise, pay attention to the shape of the back also.

Perform: 3-4 sets of 8-12 reps.

You will need: parallettes or two strong and secure parallel bars such as dumbbells with a flat bottom.

1. Grab both bars in the middle and get into the regular push-up position, making sure the bars are well rooted and sturdy.

2. Ensuring your body remains in a straight line as always, bend your elbows and slowly lower your chest downwards as far as you can comfortably go.

3. When you reach your maximum depth, push yourself back up again and to complete a rep, then repeat the process.

Beginners may not be able to get their chest to dip below their elbows. Don't force it as this may result in injury. Instead, practice this exercise regularly and you will gradually increase your range of motion. Your warm-up and preparation will also be a factor here.

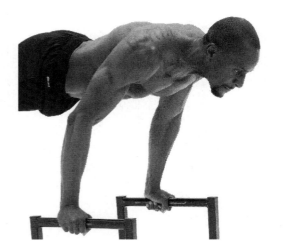
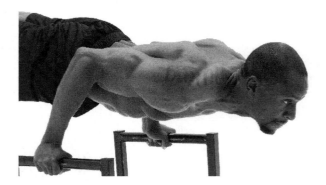

LALANNE PUSH-UP

This is a variation on the push-up with a greater emphasis on your shoulders and core. This exercise is similar to a plank, and involves maintaining tension throughout your body. Remember to control your breathing!

Perform: 2-3 sets 3-5 reps.

1. Assume the standard push-up position, with your hands under your shoulders.

2. Now walk your feet backwards, or your hands forward, until your hands are in front of your head, and you are as elongated as possible while still maintaining a straight back. Your body will start much closer to the floor than the standard push-up.

3. Keeping tension throughout your core, lower yourself until your chest touches the floor.

4. Now fire up your shoulders and core, and lift yourself back to the starting position to complete a rep.

This is something even elite calisthenics experts and personal trainers struggle with, so don't beat yourself up if it takes a long, long time to master!

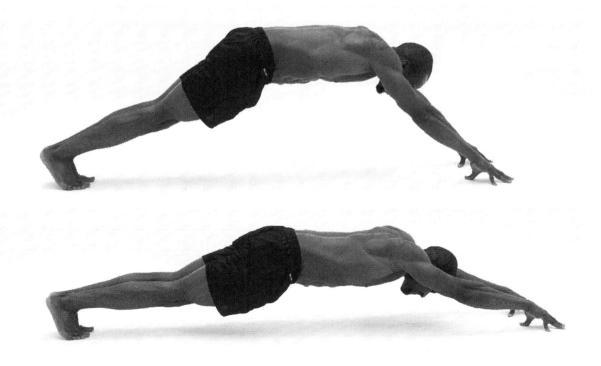

DIPS

Dips are another exercise in the 'pushing' family and are particularly good for targeting the triceps, chest and shoulders. This is another staple exercise to add to your arsenal!

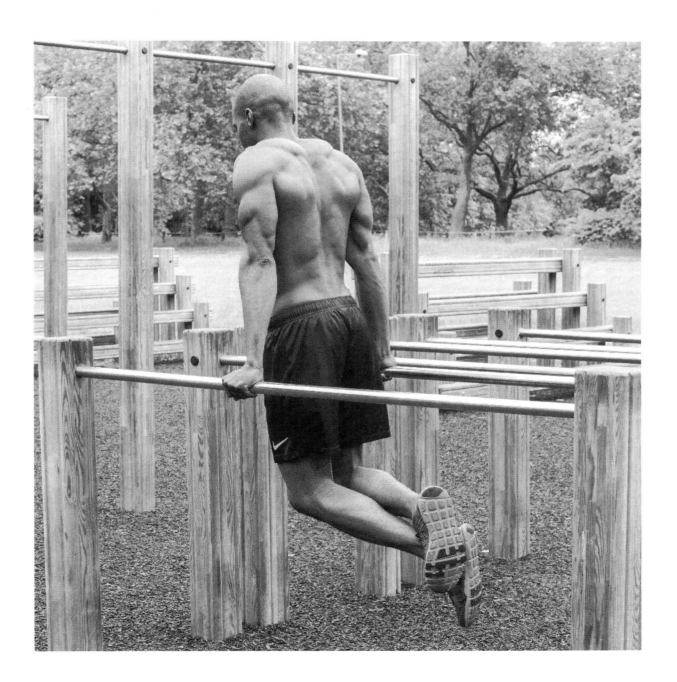

PLATFORM DIPS

This little number will get your triceps pumped and prepare you for the full version next.

Perform: 3-4 sets of 8-12 reps.

You will need: a box or sturdy raised platform.

1. With your back to the platform, place your palms on the edge and allow your fingers to rest on the front, securing your grip.

2. Stretch both legs straight out in front of you with your knees locked and rest on your heels.

3. Bend your elbows and lower yourself to the ground, keeping your back as straight and close to the platform as possible.

4. When your reach your maximum depth, push yourself back up again to complete the first rep.

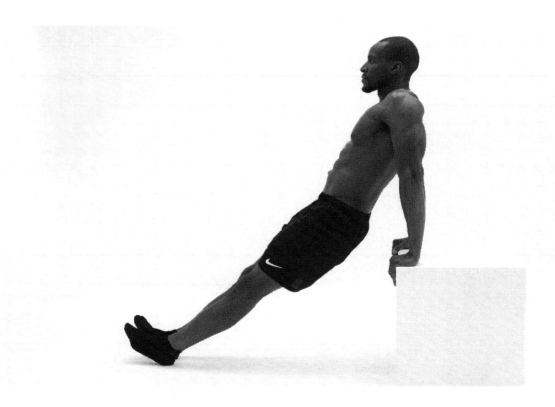

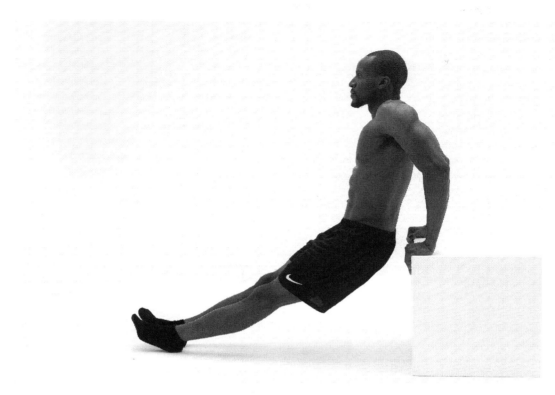

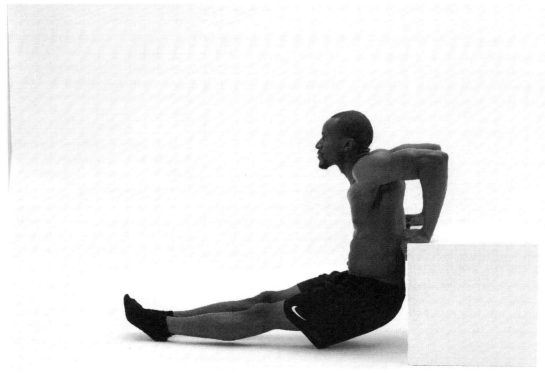

PARALLEL BAR DIPS

By lifting your feet up off the floor your are now supporting your entire bodyweight. This exercise will be tougher than the last, so remember to focus on your form and go back a step if you are finding it too difficult.

Perform: 3-4 sets of 8-12 reps.

You will need: dip station.

1. Grab the bars with your palms facing in towards your body. If your feet are touching the ground, lock them together and raise them behind you at a 90-degree angle.

2. Bend your elbows and lower yourself down as far as possible.

3. When you reach your maximum depth, push back up again and lock your elbows to complete the first rep.

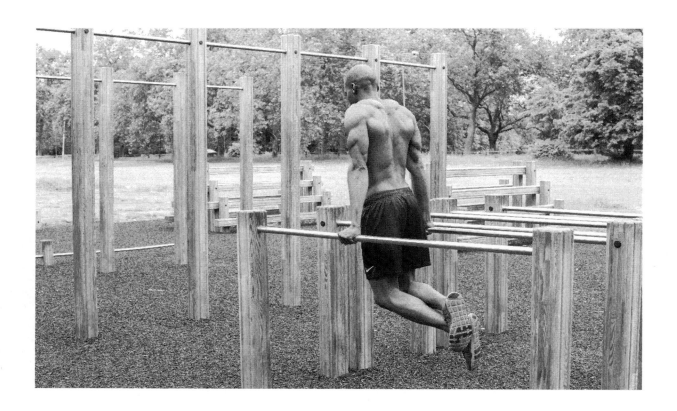

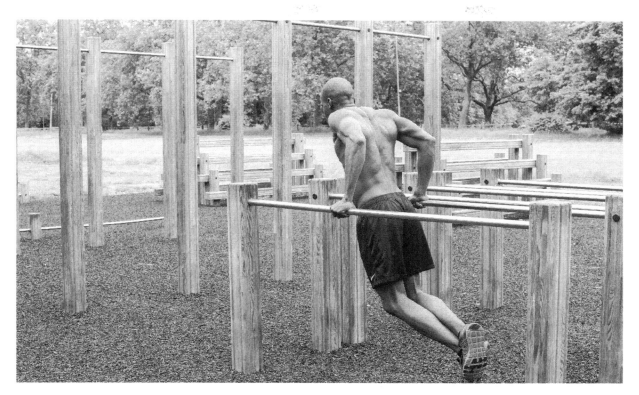

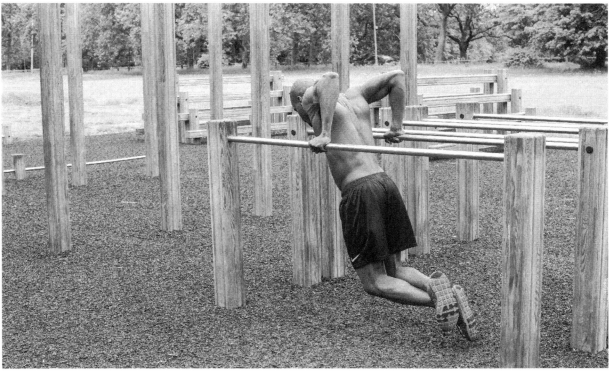

STRAIGHT BAR DIPS

This is the most difficult dip movement, so take your time and make sure you are using proper form. You might find it useful to have a spotter take some of the weight off when first training for this exercise, as it is brutally taxing on your upper body and core.

Perform: 3-4 sets of 8-12 reps.

You will need: a straight, secure bar.

1. Grab the bar with your palms facing down and hands shoulder width apart.

2. Making sure there is nothing above to bang your head on, raise yourself up until your elbows lock. This is starting position.

3. Bend your elbows and lower your body downwards. If your body / legs naturally go forwards to aid with balance, that is fine.

4. When you get as low as possible, push yourself back up until your elbows lock again to complete one rep.

NB: This exercise is a great foundation for the muscle-up, an immensely challenging exercise which combines pulling and pushing on the bar.

The muscle-up is a favorite among the calisthenics community, so it pays to train with straight bar dips in order to establish a firm foundation.

Likewise, if you find yourself struggling with the muscle-up later on, switch back to the straight bar dip to top up your pushing power.

Dips

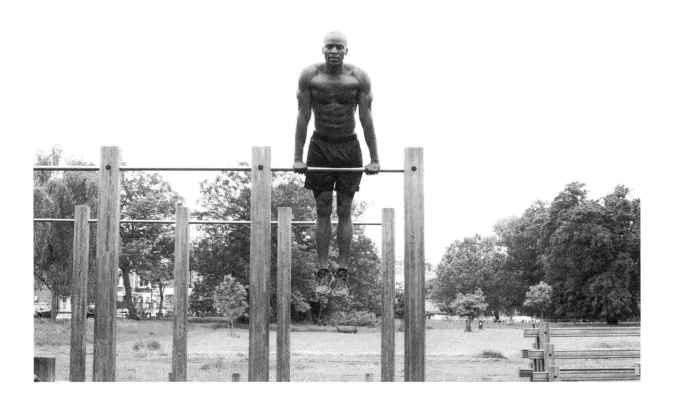

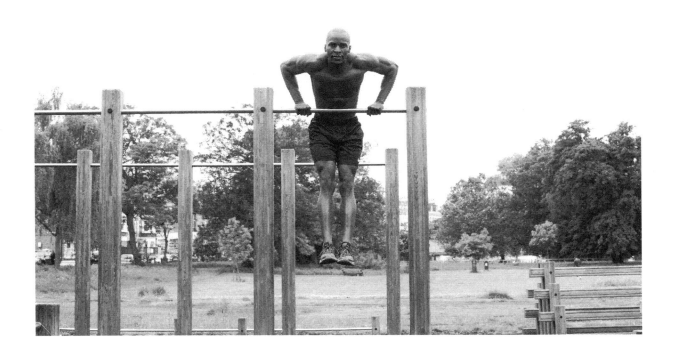

PULL-UPS / CHIN-UPS

Now that we've covered the key pushing exercises we can move on to pulling in order to target different muscle groups. Pull-ups are a complete upper body exercise that are especially good for targeting the muscles in your arms and back. Prepare for progress!

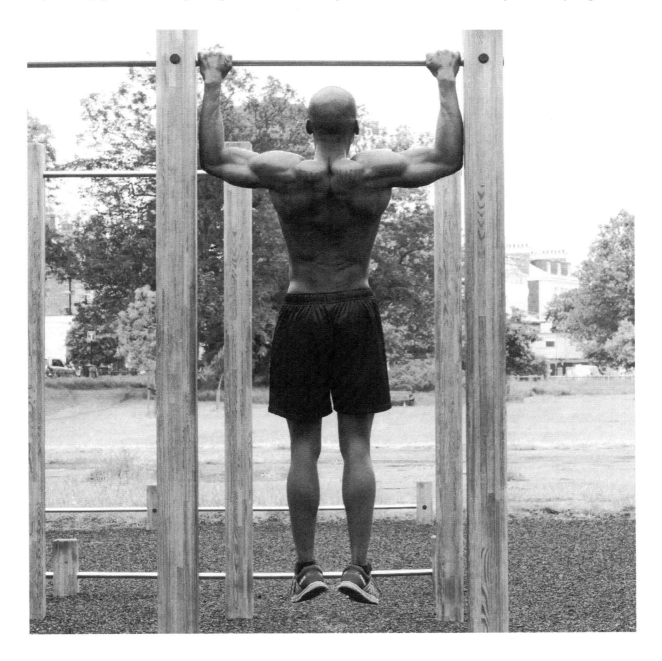

RAISED BAR ROW

This is a good place to start if you are completely new to pull-ups as, similar to raised platform push-ups, the more favorable angle makes the exercise easier to complete.

Perform: 3-4 sets of 8-12 reps.

You will need: a sturdy and secure bar.

1. Grab the bar with an overhand grip and straighten your arms.

2. Walk your legs forward in front of the bar so your body is at an angle (the greater the angle, the more difficult the exercise.) This is start position.

3. Ensuring your body stays straight and your feet remain in position, pull your chest up until it touches the bar.

4. When your chest has touched the bar or gone as far as possible, lower yourself back down and straighten your arms to complete one rep.

Variations:

• Move the bar up to make the exercise easier, or down to make it harder.

• Use TRX straps instead of a bar.

• Use an underhand grip.

• Move your hands closer / further apart.

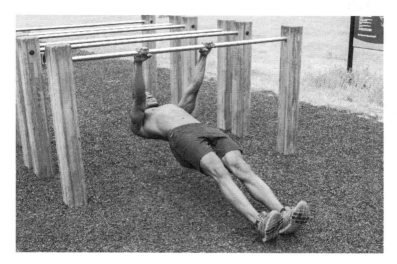

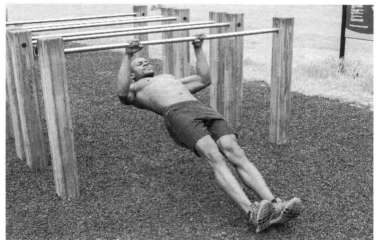

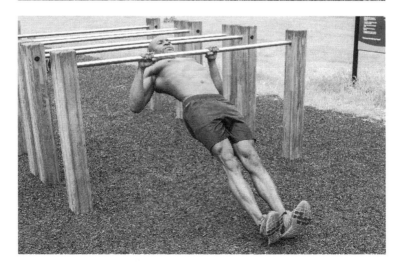

NEGATIVE CHIN-UP

Chin-ups can be an intimidating exercise to master but fortunately, as with most other calisthenics exercises, there is a simpler variation you can try first.

Perform: 3-4 sets of 3-5 reps.

You will need: a pull-up bar.

1. Get to the top position of a chin-up, using a platform, spotter or simply jumping if you can't quite make it under your own steam.

2. Slowly lower yourself down, tensing your muscles to work them as much as possible, until your arms are straight and elbows are locked, then drop off the bar to complete one rep and reset.

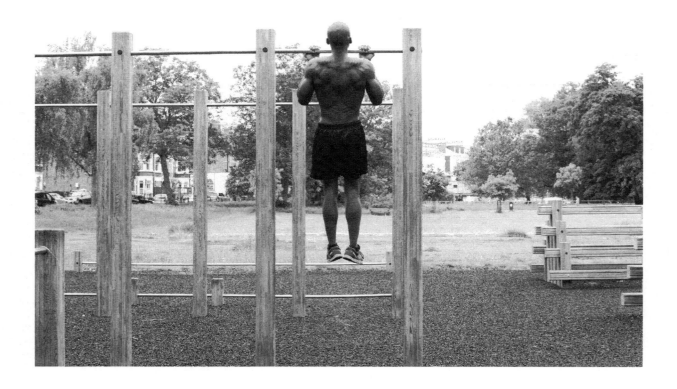

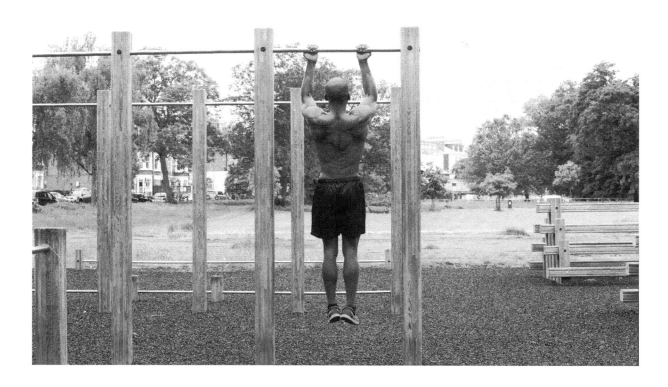

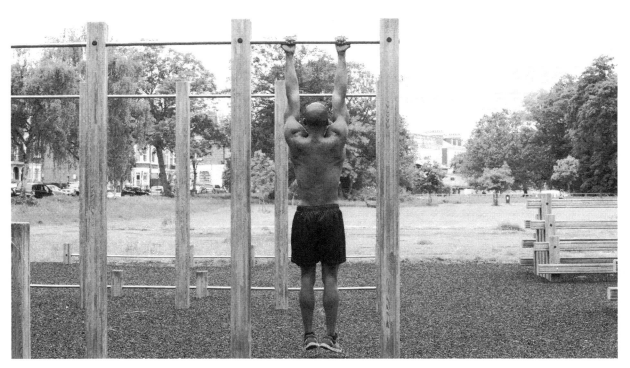

STATIC HOLD

Another simple variation on the pull-up is one that requires no movement at all in order to build the strength required to dive into the full version.

Perform: 20 second hold time.

You will need: a pull-up bar.

1. Achieve the position you wish to hold by pulling, jumping, using a box or lowering yourself into it.

2. Lock your muscles in place and try to hold this position for the allotted time.

3. Once complete, slowly lower yourself down and drop off the bar. If you don't quite complete the allotted time, throw in as many sets as it takes to reach that total amount e.g. 2x 10 seconds = 20 seconds.

NB: This differs from the negative chin-up in that you will be spending as much time as possible holding your position to build strength and endurance.

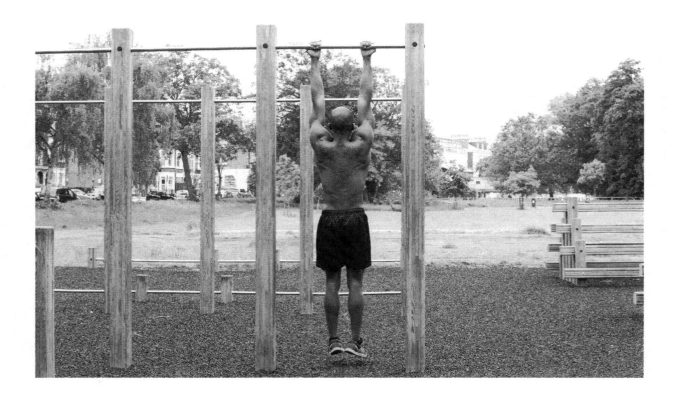

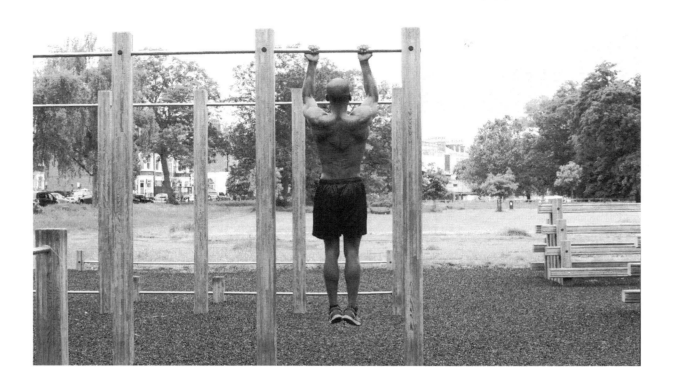

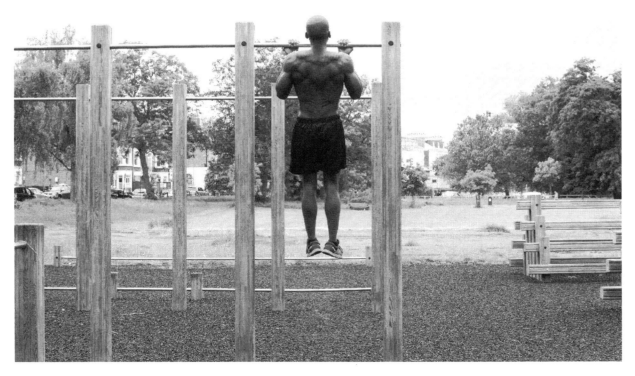

CHIN-UP

Once you can comfortably perform the introductory exercises you can move onto the real thing! Chin-ups are the easiest of the full bodyweight pulling exercises as they leverage the two muscle groups that tend to already be strongest; the biceps and chest.

That said this can still be difficult for beginners so remember to focus on your form and go with quality over quantity!

Perform: 3-4 sets of 8-12 reps.

You will need: a pull-up bar.

1. Using an underhand grip, grab the bar with your hands approximately shoulder width apart.

2. Relax your shoulders, allowing them to sag down. Lock your elbows and lift your feet up so you are hanging freely. This is your starting position.

3. Pull your body up as high as possible, the aim being to get your chin above the bar or have your chest touch against it. Do not swing your body or legs or use momentum to help you.

4. When you reach the top position, lower yourself back down slowly and hang freely again to complete the first rep.

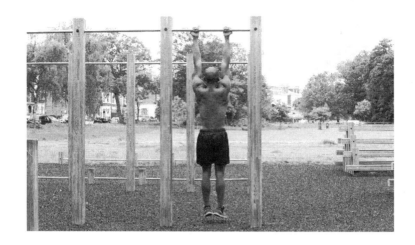

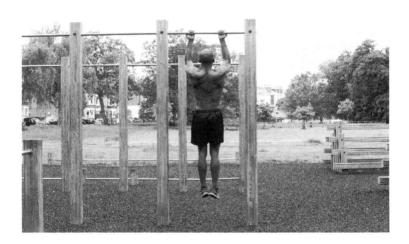

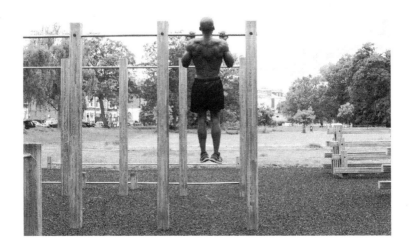

PULL-UP

This exercise essentially follows the same formula as the chin-up, but with one crucial difference; overhand instead of underhand grip.

By changing to this grip you are taking away much of the biceps' ability to assist with the lift, effectively transferring that effort and energy to your back, specifically the lats.

Again, feel free to perform rows, negatives and statics in order to build your way up to this exercise.

Perform: 3-4 sets of 8-12 reps.

You will need: a pull-up bar.

1. Grab the pull-up bar using an overhand grip with your hands approximately shoulder width apart.

2. Lift your feet off the ground and hang with your elbows locked straight to achieve start position.

3. Keeping your legs and body straight and without using momentum, pull yourself up towards the bar until your chin is above it or your chest is touching it.

4. From here, lower yourself down to the start position to complete one rep.

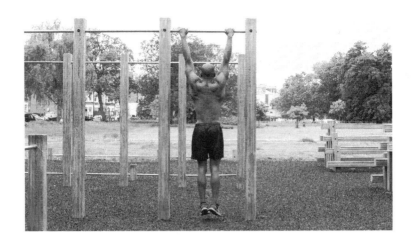

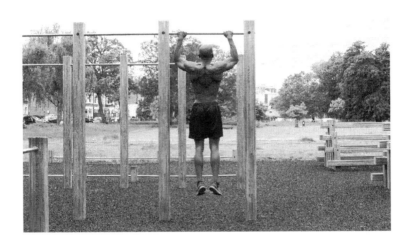

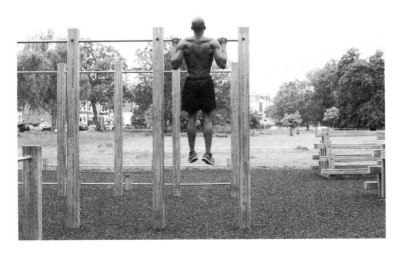

CLOSE GRIP PULL-UP

This is a simple variation on the pull-up that will bring variety to your upper body work-out by targeting slightly different areas of the arms and back.

Perform: 3-4 sets of 8-12 reps.

You will need: a pull-up bar.

1. Grab the pull-up bar using an overhand grip with your hands close together.

2. Lift your feet off the ground and hang with your elbows locked straight. You're ready to get started now.

3. Keeping your legs and body straight and without using momentum, pull yourself up towards the bar until your chin is above it or your chest is touching it.

4. From here, lower yourself down to the start position to complete one rep.

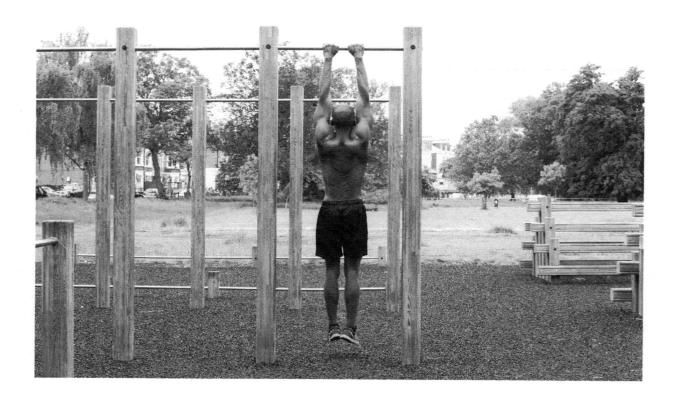

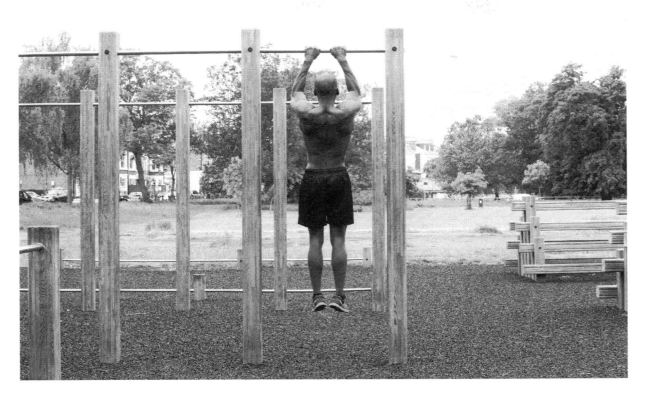

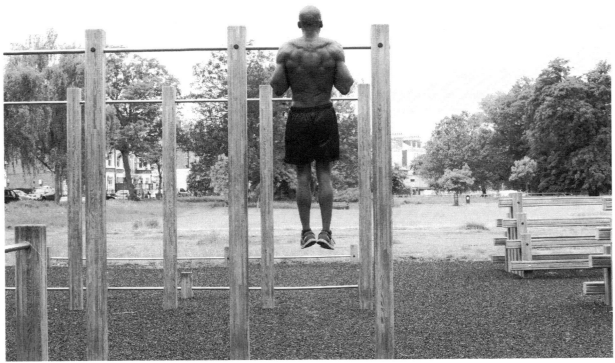

WIDE GRIP PULL-UP

Effectively the opposite of the previous exercise, this is one that will really test your back strength. Both can also be done in chin-up form.

Perform: 3-4 sets of 8-12 reps.

You will need: a pull-up bar.

1. Grab the pull-up bar using an overhand grip with your hands close together.

2. As you now know, lift your feet off the ground and hang with your elbows locked straight to get into the starting position.

3. Keeping your legs and body straight and without using momentum, pull yourself up towards the bar until your chin is above it or your chest is touching it.

4. Lower down to the start position to complete one rep. Go straight into the next rep.

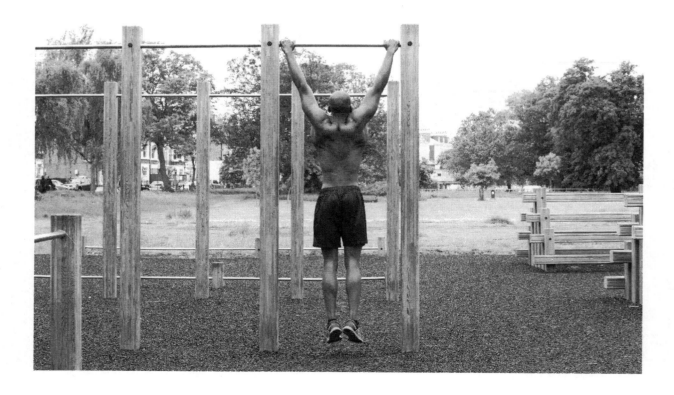

Pull-Ups / Chin-Ups

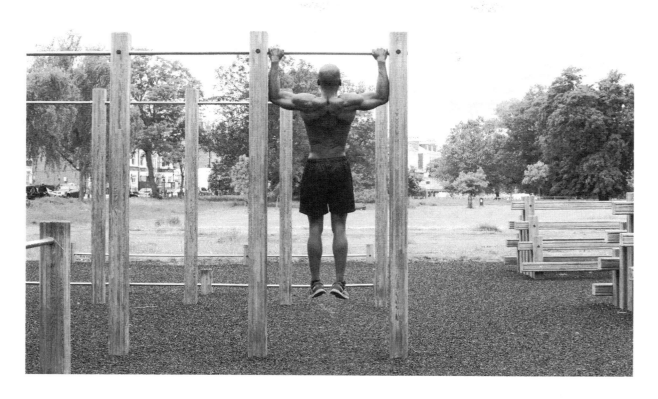

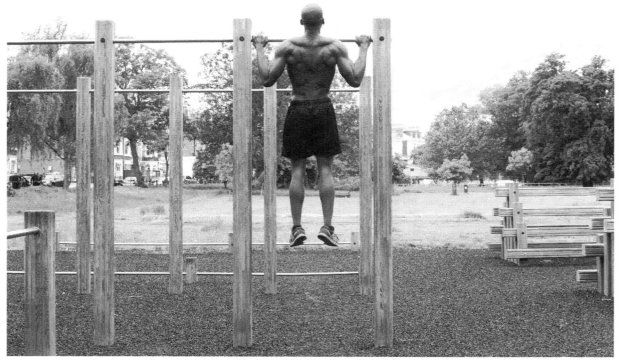

CLAP PULL-UP

This explosive movement is sure to push your strength to the limits! Like the clap push-up we are introducing a quick, explosive movement to an otherwise slow and controlled motion to spice up the movement and keep your body guessing. Let the fun begin!

Perform: 3-4 sets of 3-4 reps.

You will need: pull-up bar.

1. Assume the standard pull-up position with your hands directly over your shoulders, grasping the bar with an overhand grip, hanging freely.

2. Ensure your arms are completely locked out, and pull up as forcefully and powerfully as you can. Imagine trying to shoot yourself through the roof!

3. Just as your chin passes the bar, take your hands off and perform a quick clap in front of your chest.

4. The same instant you complete the clap, whip your hands back onto the bar and grab it on your descent, returning to start position to complete 1 rep.

It's a good idea to practice this with something soft to land on, as you may find it takes a little time to build up the reaction speed and strength required to catch the bar.

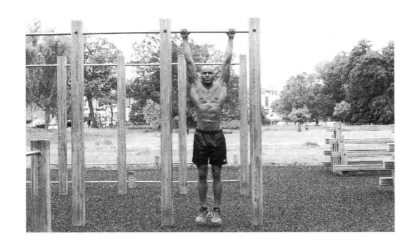

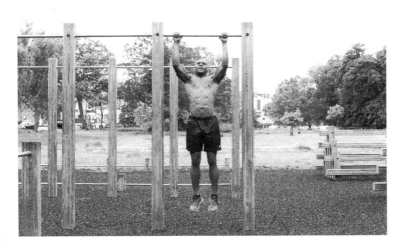

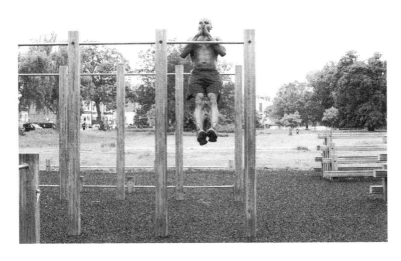

REAR PULL-UP

This is a perfect example of how a slight change in orientation can make a movement more difficult and work your muscles in an entirely new way.

Perform: 3-4 sets of 8-12 reps.

You Will Need: a pull-up bar.

1. Grab the bar as you would for a standard pull-up; overhand, approximately shoulder width apart, or slightly more, hanging freely.

2. Start at the bottom with your arms completely straight, and begin to pull yourself up towards the bar in a slow, controlled, movement.

3. As you are pulling up, pull your scapulae (or shoulder blades) back and lean your head forward slightly.

4. At the top of the movement, the bar should be behind your neck and just touching the top of your shoulders. Be careful not to bang it against the bar. Wrap a towel around your shoulders if need be.

5. Slowly lower yourself back down to finish a rep.

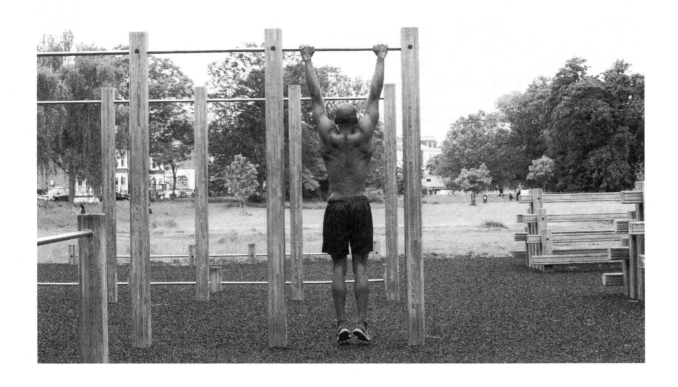

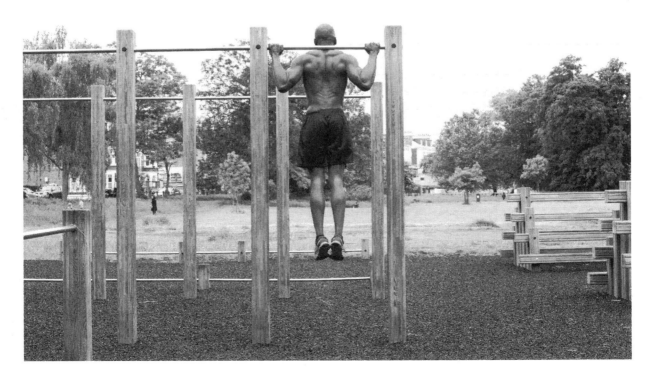

FINGERTIPS PULL-UP

A superb exercise for all those climbers out there! This form of the pull-up is essentially identical to the standard pull-up, except we'll be using the fingers to grip the bar and not our entire hands.

Perform: 3-4 sets of 3-5 reps.

You will need: a pull-up bar.

1. Take up the standard pull-up position, but apply the grip with only your fingers. We recommend starting with four fingers, leaving out your thumb from the grip, gradually reducing them as you get more comfortable.

There's no need to show the whole motion over again with photos, but just in case you need a reminder, follow the below progression:

2. Ensure you are hanging freely with your arms completely locked out to start, and begin to pull yourself up.

3. Once your chin is above the bar, slowly lower yourself to the starting position to finish your first rep. As always, go straight into the next with controlled movement.

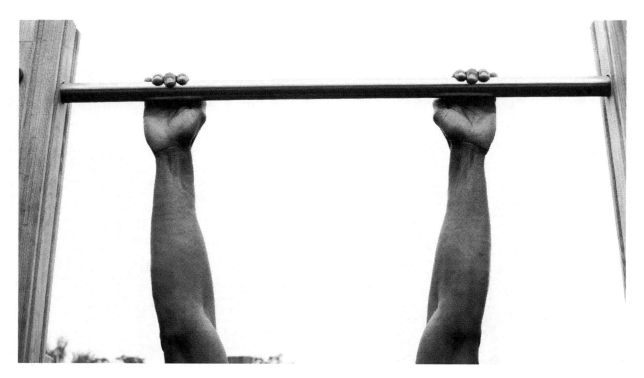

ROCK CLIMBER PULL-UP

Here we essentially have the pull-up version of the archer push-up. We'll primarily be working the strength of one arm at a time, while using the other for stability and a little extra force.

Perform: 3 sets of 3-6 reps per side.

You will need: a pull-up bar.

1. Grasp the bar with the standard overhand grip, but spread your hands so your grip is as wide as you can manage. Hang freely to start.

2. Pull yourself up towards one hand, while straightening out the other arm.

3. Once at the top, lower back to the start point. This counts as 1 rep for that side. Now pull yourself up to the other hand and repeat.

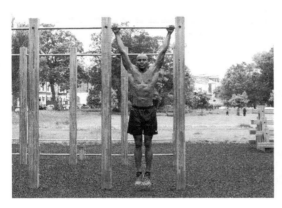
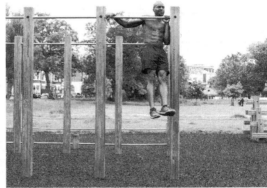
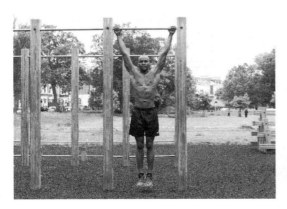
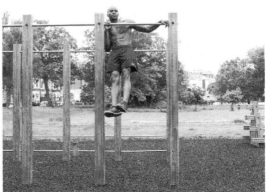

L PULL-UP

This version of the pull-up is a complete package, with work for your quads, core, back, shoulders, chest and arms! Your legs and core will be maintaining tension throughout the course of the maneuver while you engage your back, arms, chest and shoulders to lift your body.

Perform: 3-4 sets of 8-12 reps.

You will need: a pull-up bar.

1. Assume the standard pull-up position with your hands a little wider apart than your shoulders, grasping the bar with an overhand grip.

2. Lift up your legs until they are parallel with the ground. Ensure that your legs are completely straight from hip to heel. This is your starting position.

3. Now engage your back and shoulders to pull your chin over the bar, while maintaining your straight legs.

4. Once your chin is above the bar, lower yourself down to the starting position while maintaining straight legs. That's one rep done!

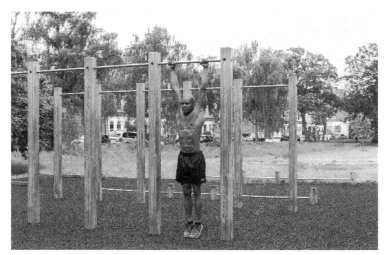

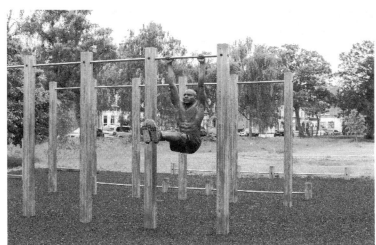

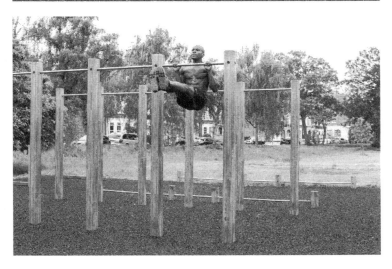

STRAIGHT LINE PULL-UP

This little-known variation of the pull-up targets your biceps, shoulders and lats and is a great way to make extra use of one simple piece of equipment.

Perform: 3 sets of 8-12 reps.

You will need: a pull-up bar.

1. Position yourself underneath the bar so that it is running in the same direction that you are looking.

2. Grasp the bar with both hands, with the palms facing each other. Your hands should be touching.

3. Loosen up your shoulders and shrug them down, lean back just enough so you're looking up at the bar, feet slightly off the ground to start with.

4. Begin to pull yourself up and raise your chest until it's touching the bar. If your bar posts are tight together so you cannot lean back enough, try lifting until your shoulder hits the bar as shown.

5. Now lower yourself back to the start point to complete your rep.

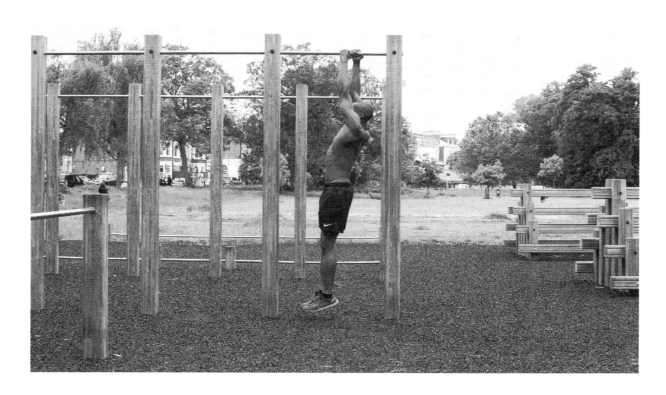

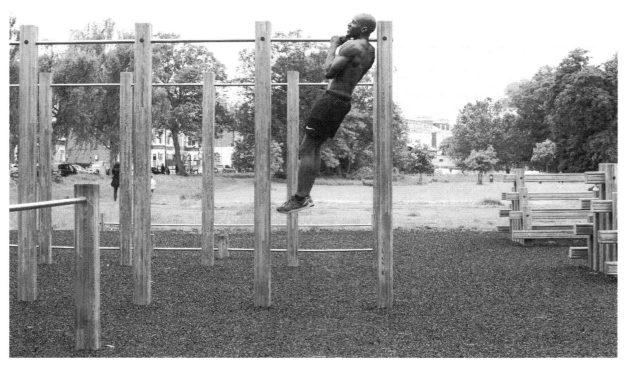

PARALLEL PULL-UP

This is the perfect variation of the pull-up to challenge both your arms and core. You will be maintaining full tension through your core and back, while firing your arms and shoulders for the pull-up. This is an ideal movement to prep your core for several of the lever movements that we will cover later.

Perform: 3-4 sets of 3-5 reps.

You will need: a pull-up bar.

1. Assume the standard pull-up position with your hands grasping the bar in an overhand grip.

2. Begin to pull yourself up, firing your core, glutes, and back at the same time to orient your body parallel to the ground so you're looking upwards.

3. Continue to pull yourself up, and endeavor to get your chest as close to the bar as you can.

4. Once you have reached the top of the movement, stay horizontal and lower yourself in a slow, controlled, motion until your arms are locked out. One rep, nailed!

Variation: If you struggle to perform the pull-up once in the parallel position, try tucking your legs in as shown. This is a great starting place. Extend your legs out as and when you become stronger.

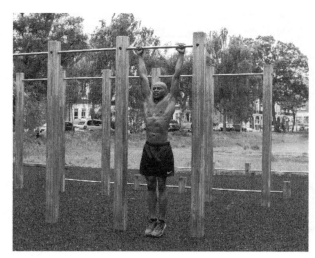 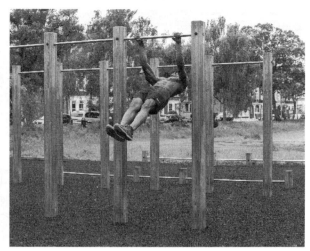

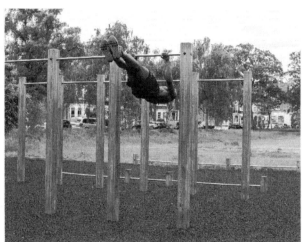 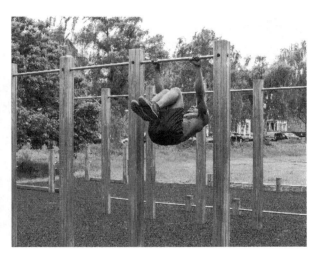

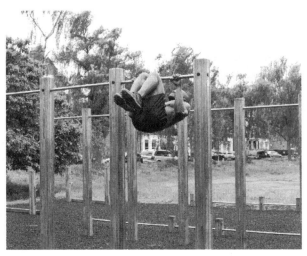

TYPEWRITER PULL-UP

This may look a lot like the rock climber pull-up, but it differs in that you are gliding left and right across the bar, rather than pulling up to the left or right from the bottom position.

Perform: 3-4 sets of 3-5 reps.

You will need: a pull-up bar.

1. Grip the bar overhand, with your hands wide apart.

2. Starting from the hanging position, with arms fully extended, perform a standard wide grip pull-up until your chin is above the bar. Hold it there.

3. Slowly pull yourself to your right hand while straightening out your left arm. Ensure that your chin stays above the bar.

4. Your hands should not change position, but your grip on your left hand will shift from an overhand grip to a looser grip that is simply bracing your body. Your left arm should lock out as much as the bar width allows and help support your body.

5. Once you have reached as far to the right as possible, slowly shift back to the middle, while keeping your chin above the bar, and then repeat to the left. A complete cycle counts as 1 repetition.

As your strength and control over the movement increases, begin to gradually increase the number of reps you perform.

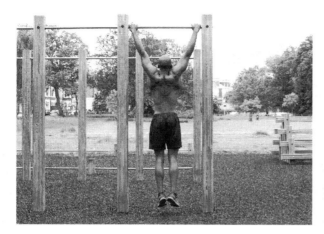
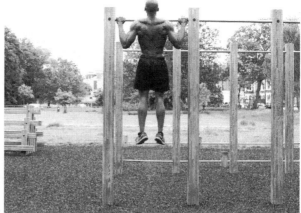

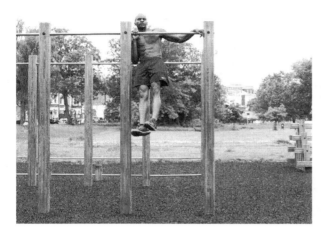
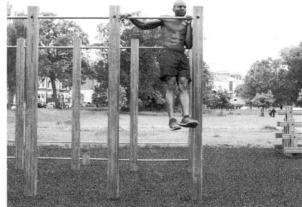

FINGER ASSIST SINGLE-ARM PULL-UP

As you progress towards a strict one-arm pull-up, this exercise will enable you to limit the assistance you get from your other hand, eventually eliminating it completely.

Perform: 3-4 sets of 3-5 reps on each arm.

You will need: a pull-up bar.

1. Assume the standard pull-up position, with only one hand using the complete overhand grip. The other hand should be gripping the bar with 1-4 fingers.

2. Ensure that your arms are fully locked out, and then begin to pull yourself up. Try to use your supporting hand only as needed.

3. Once your chin is over the bar, slowly lower yourself back down to finish the rep.

Reduce the number of fingers you use on your supporting hand as your strength builds.

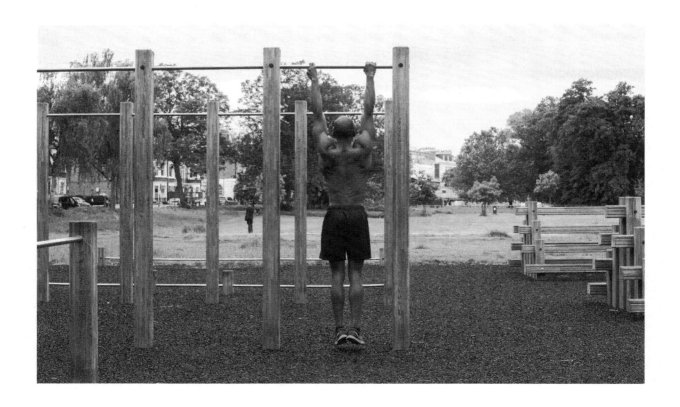

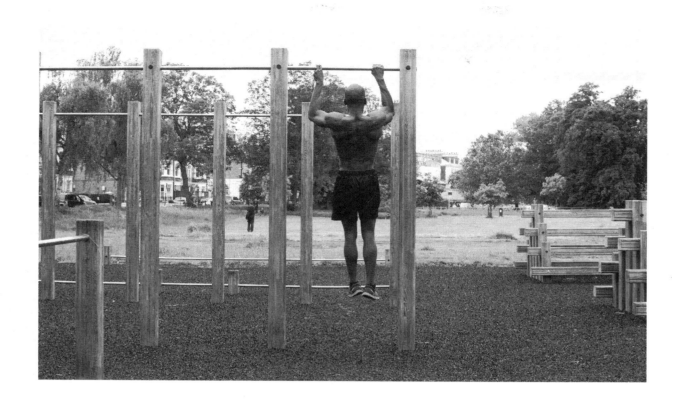

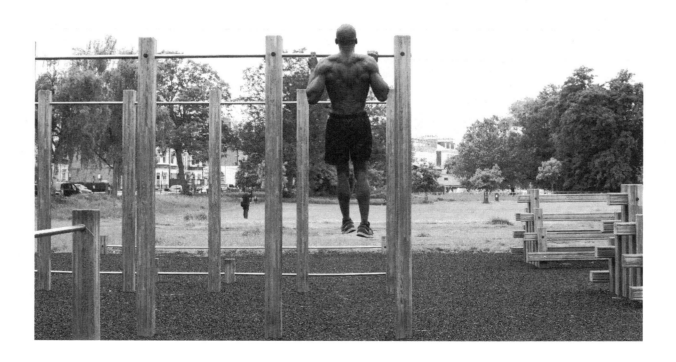

ASSISTED SINGLE-ARM PULL-UP

A rope or towel can also help you on your way to the one-arm pull-up. In this case we'll only be using the towel for one hand, while the hand gripping the bar will perform the lion's share of the work.

Perform: 3-4 sets of 3-5 reps on each arm.

You will need: a pull-up bar.

1. Drape a towel over the bar and bring the ends together. Now assume pull-up position with one hand gripping the towel, and the other using an underhand grip on the bar.

2. From a fully extended position, begin to pull yourself up with the arm that's gripping the bar, and only use the towel hand as needed for support.

3. Once your chin is above the bar, slowly lower yourself back to the start position. This is 1 complete rep.

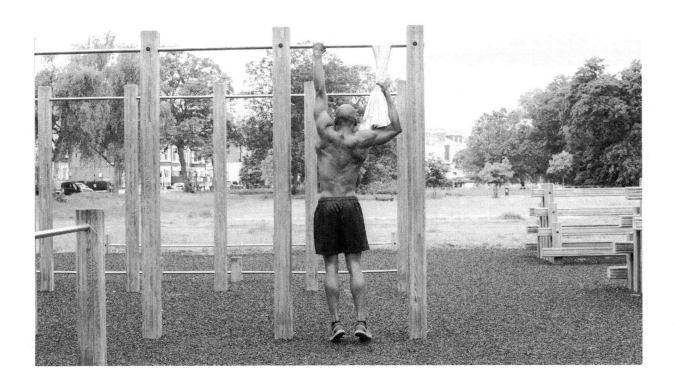

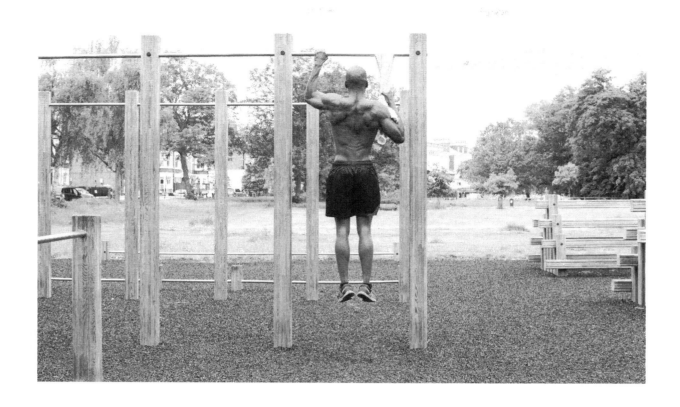

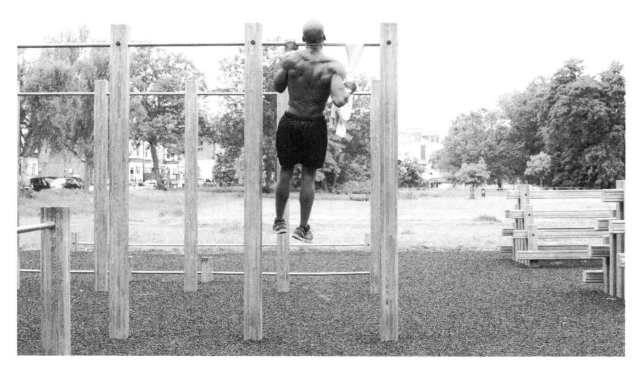

COMPLETE SINGLE-ARM PULL-UP

If you've reached the stage where you can complete all the recommended sets and reps for single-arm exercises so far, then it's time for the big game! The single-arm pull-up is incredibly challenging, as you've no doubt discovered already. However, its strength building qualities are phenomenal and well worth the struggle!

Perform: 2-3 sets of 3-5 reps per arm.

You will need: a pull-up bar.

1. Stand under the bar and locate your hand directly over your head. Grasp the bar with an underhand grip.

2. Start with your arm fully locked out, and begin the movement by firing your shoulder, and pulling your scapula down.

3. Now pull with everything you've got, and raise your chin over the bar.

4. Slowly lower yourself back to the starting position to complete 1 repetition.

Variations: Remember, negatives and statics can help build up the strength required to reach this stage!

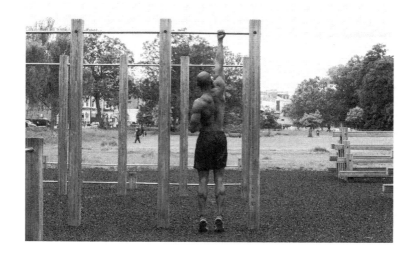

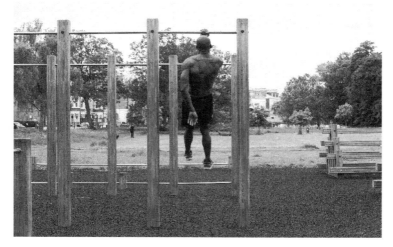

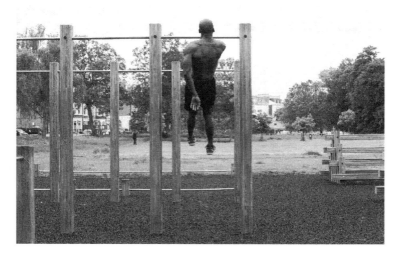

HANGING PULL-UP

Not got a training rope? Grab that sweat towel again and prepare to improve your grip with this innovative exercise. Just make sure it can take your weight first!

You may find it useful to have a spotter hold your feet in place when first learning this exercise, as you will have a tendency to twist and spin around which will detract your attention from using the proper form.

Ask your buddy to gently take a hold of your ankles to stop any swaying, so that you can focus fully on hauling yourself towards the bar!

Perform: 3-4 sets of 3-5 reps.

You will need: pull-up bar and rope / sweat towel.

1. Drape the towel over the bar and bring the ends together.

2. Grip both ends of the towel in each hand, and hang with your arms completely locked out for your starting position.

3. In a continuous, controlled movement, pull yourself up until your hands are about level with the center of your chest.

4. Now lower yourself back to the starting position to complete one repetition.

Variation: If you can complete most or all of the pull-up variations we have presented so far, then add a little extra weight for a greater challenge. Simply use a weighted vest, dip belt, or kettlebell / dumbbell between the feet while performing the movements.

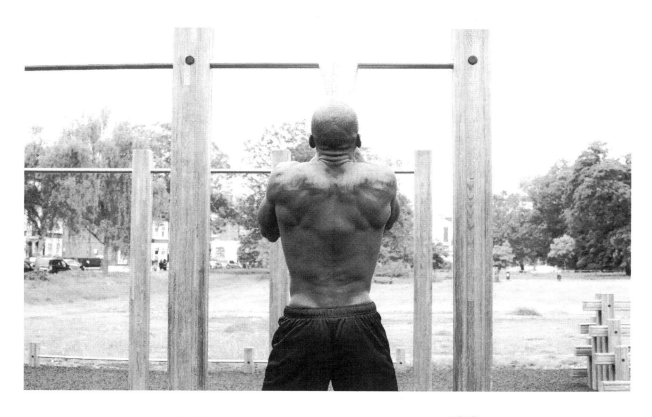

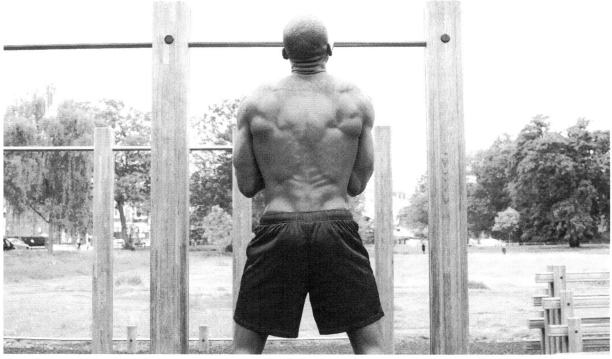

MUSCLE-UPS

When you are comfortable with all variations of the pushing and pulling exercises we've presented on the bar up to this point then you are ready to take on a truly versatile and astonishingly effective combination of both. Prepare for war, comrade, this one's tough!

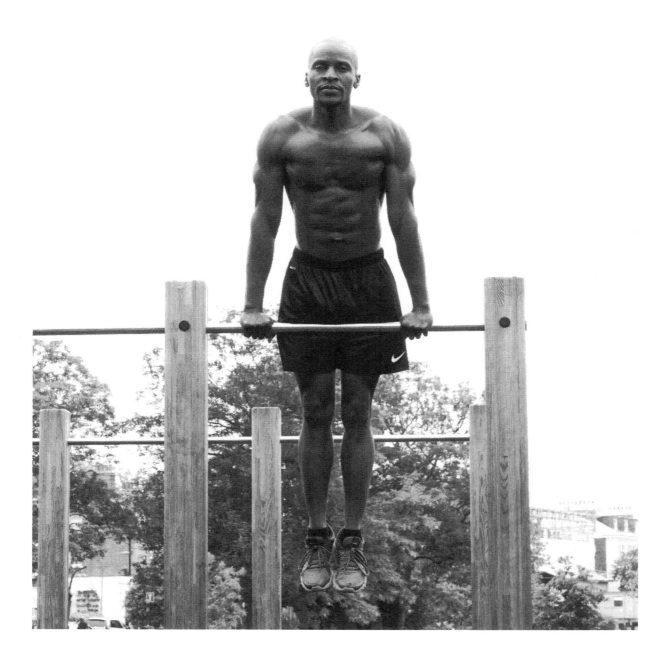

STANDARD MUSCLE-UP

There is nothing 'standard' about the amount of strength required to perform this one without swinging around like a safari park chimp. Work up to it and you will get there!

Perform: 3-4 sets of 6-10 reps.

You will need: a pull-up bar.

1. Grab that bar using an overhand grip, hands approximately shoulder width apart.

2. Perform a pull-up, hauling yourself up to the bar with as much power as possible.

3. In one movement, loosen your grip slightly, rotate your hands forward so you can prepare to push in the second step (see the false grip next for more).

4. Without stopping, push yourself up as high as possible, locking your elbows at the top of the movement.

5. Perform the process in reverse to lower yourself back down and complete 1 rep. Do not drop off the bar.

Variations:

• If you are struggling to generate enough power to bring your chin above the bar, you can use your feet for a little added momentum. At step 2, swing your feet forward very slightly, and then use the backwards momentum which follows to pull yourself up to the bar with as much power as possible.

• You can also practice each part individually and then piece them together over time to make it simpler.

This exercise will take a lot of practice – the aim is to complete the whole thing in one fluid motion without using momentum, so don't rely on that to get by.

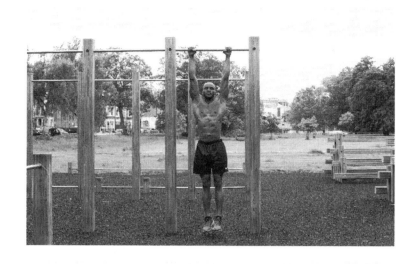

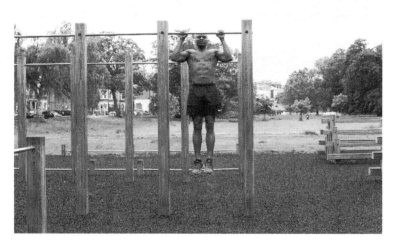

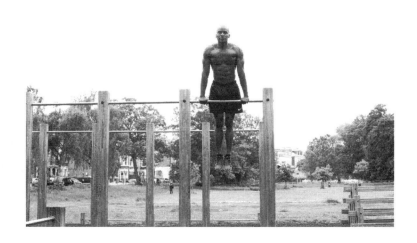

FALSE GRIP HANG

The forthcoming variation will require a great deal of explosive strength and quick movements on the pull-up bar. To increase control over this movement, we'll first go over the fundamental grip that will be used. This is the same grip you should previously have used to transition from pulling to pushing in the standard muscle-up.

Perform: 3-5 sets of 5-10 second holds.

You will need: pull-up bar.

1. Standing under the bar, place the base of your palms against it.

2. Bring your fingers down and grip the bar as best as you can without losing your palm placement. You may only be able to get your fingertips to the front of the bar, which is fine. The idea is to have a secure yet fluid grip that allows for a smooth transition.

3. Now practice hanging from this grip until you become comfortable with it.

4. Once you are comfortable with hanging, move onto the full movement next.

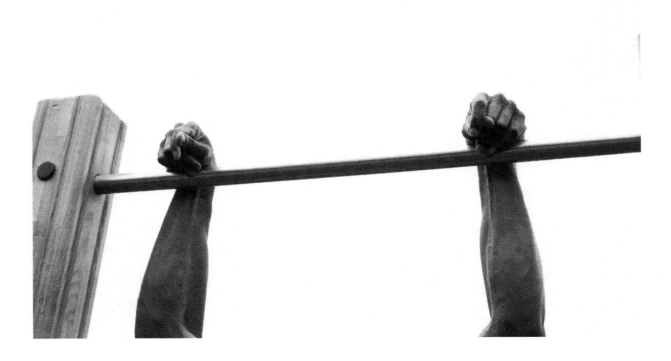

FALSE GRIP MUSCLE-UP

When you have reached the point where the false grip is comfortable, or at the very least manageable, then it's time to add in the muscle-up. This is an exceptionally taxing movement, and takes a great deal of control. Move slowly and don't push the pace! Take time to build up your strength and master the form to perfection.

The mechanics of this exercise are exactly the same as the standard muscle-up, only with the change in grip as shown previously, so simply refer back to the previous two sets of photos to see how it should be done, and follow the below instructions.

Perform: 3-4 sets of 3-5 reps.

You will need: pull-up bar.

1. Grip the bar with the false grip that we have already covered, with your hands around shoulder width apart. Take up a dead hang with your arms locked out.

2. Slowly begin to pull yourself up. Do not try and launch yourself upwards. Always stay in control!

3. As your chin passes the bar, roll your shoulders forward, and pull forcibly to get your shoulders over the bar.

4. Once your shoulders pass your hands, transition and push down on the bar as hard as you can to push yourself up until your arms are straight.

5. Once your arms are completely straight over the bar, slowly lower yourself back to the starting position to complete 1 rep.

HANDSTANDS

Consider the strength your legs must possess to carry you around all day, and now think about how great it would be if you could transfer that level of strength to the upper body, too. This is exactly what we aim to achieve through handstand exercises. Let's go!

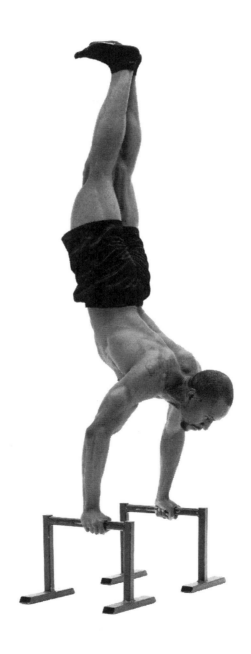

WALL WALKS

If you haven't performed a handstand recently or even at all then this is the perfect exercise to build up your strength at the same time as your confidence.

You should be somewhat familiar with this exercise from the wall push-ups presented previously. The difference here is that we'll be taking it up a little higher and transferring a greater load to the shoulders, arms and hands in prep for performing handstands.

Perform: maximum hold time possible.

You will need: a solid wall that can take your weight.

1. Get into a regular push-up position but instead of placing your feet on the floor, place them flat against the bottom of the wall.

2. Keeping your arms and legs as straight as possible and your core pulled in tight, begin to walk your feet up the wall in small steps. As they get higher you will also need to move your hands backwards to support your bodyweight.

3. When you have walked up as high as possible, aim to hold this position for a few seconds before slowly walking back down to the start, again aiming to keep your arms, legs and body straight.

As your strength and confidence increases you can walk higher and extend the amount of time you hold the top position.

Super important: This is a nice, gentle introduction to being upside-down, but can still be quite disorientating.

Take it slow, and at the first sign of dizziness or discomfort, come down and stay seated for a little while until you regain your composure. Don't try to stand up or jump straight into another exercise after being upside-down, as your body needs time to adjust.

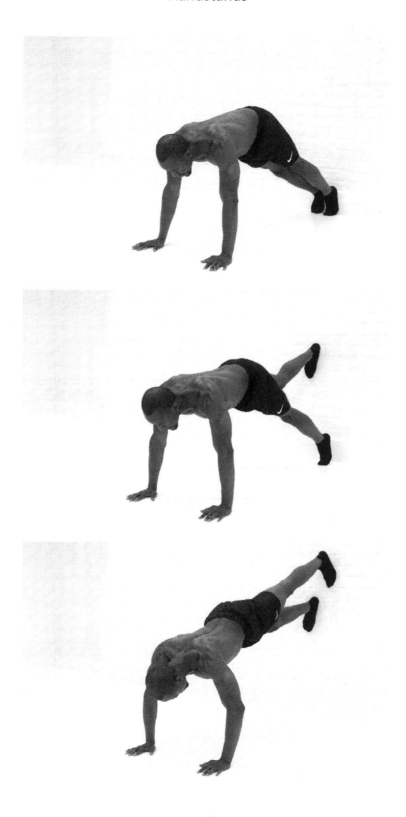

WALL SUPPORT HANDSTAND

Not to be confused with wall walks, this is the next step in the progression of handstand exercises. This time, instead of walking up the wall you will 'kick' up against it in order to get into position.

Perform: maximum hold time possible.

You will need: a solid wall, which can take your weight and a spotter if you're new to this (just don't kick them in the face!)

1. Facing the wall, place your hands shoulder width apart on the floor, approximately a foot away from the wall and spread your fingers out wide for balance.

2. Get into 'starting block' pose by tucking one leg up close to your chest and extending the other out behind you. There is no right or wrong foot here, simply find what works for you or switch it up as and when you please.

3. Use the leg that is tucked underneath you to kick upwards while swinging the back leg over with the momentum generated. This should be enough to get you into the wall supported handstand position if you commit to it.

If you are nervous about performing this step, try kicking up small amounts at first. When you are ready to go for it, commit with confidence that the wall WILL catch you, or use a spotter if necessary.

4. When you are in the handstand position, hold it for as long as possible, keeping your whole body locked straight. Stay calm and breathe normally.

5. To descend, keep your arms locked and drop one leg followed by the other. Try to control this movement rather than simply dropping down like a sack of spuds as this will build even greater strength.

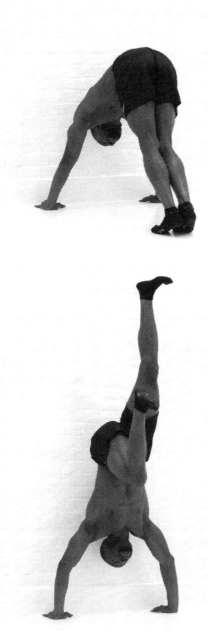

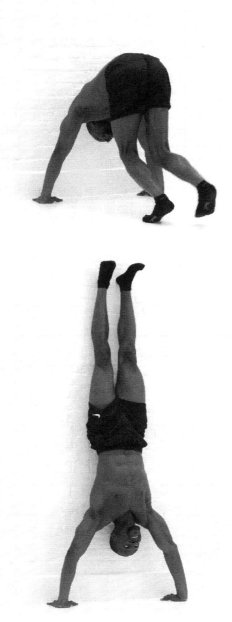

WALL HANDSTAND TO FREE HANDSTAND

Once you're comfortable with wall-supported handstands, it's time to begin the process of moving away from the wall to develop your balance.

Perform: maximum hold time possible.

You will need: a solid wall that can take your weight and a spotter if you're new to this (again try not to hit them on your way up!)

1. Kick up into a wall handstand and remain there.

2. With as much force as possible, push down with your fingertips to encourage your feet away from the wall. If this doesn't work, push away from the wall VERY softly with your feet.

3. When your feet are no longer touching the wall try to balance in this position for as long as possible. If you find yourself falling back towards the wall, or overbalancing, correct this by pushing down hard with your fingertips. If you experience the opposite, under-balancing, try bending your elbows a little and engaging your shoulders to assist.

4. Hold the handstand for as long as possible. If you fall back into the wall or down to the floor, simply get back into position and try again. Remember, your feet should stay together and come away from the wall as shown.

NB: The biggest obstacle to performing this exercise can often be mental. Fear of failure or injury often causes us to be indecisive, but you needn't be concerned with this if you are in a safe environment and / or have a spotter with you.

Trust in your own preparation and, even if you do fall back down, it will be a controlled descent. Don't forget to spend a few moments regaining your composure before getting up to perform another exercise!

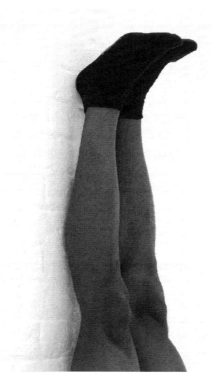

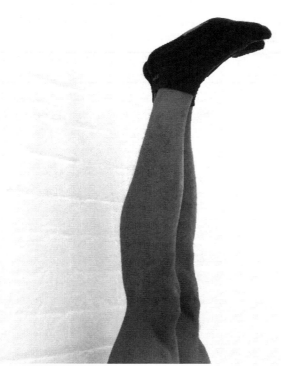

HANDSTAND BAILOUT

Before you dive into free handstands it is important to learn how to recover if you begin to topple over. Once you have mastered this move, you will be able to take on free handstands without the need for a spotter.

Perform: as many repetitions as needed to feel confident.

You will need: an open space and matted flooring if possible.

1. Kick up into a handstand (or attempt to!)

2. When you go into overbalance – that is your legs and feet going over your head – take one hand off the floor. By doing this you will cause your body to pivot around the hand that is still rooted to the floor. People normally choose to keep their strongest hand rooted but find what works best for you.

3. Allow the momentum generated to bring your body around, and then place the hand you lifted up back to the floor and let your legs come back down safely.

Practice this technique until it becomes a reflex and you will never again have to suffer the pain or embarrassment of going down like a Jenga tower!

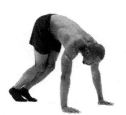 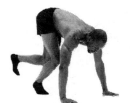 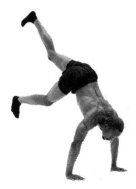

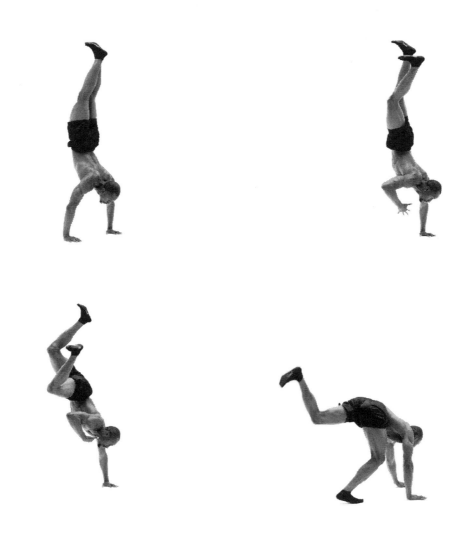

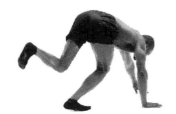

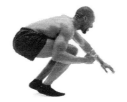

FLOOR / FREE HANDSTAND

The final stage of the standard handstand is the free handstand. Don't worry if this seems daunting at first – you have your escape strategy so you'll be able to bail out if things don't go to plan right away.

Perform: maximum hold time possible.

You will need: a clear space and matted flooring if possible.

1. Ensuring there is plenty of room around you, kick up into a handstand.

2. Your feet will likely travel over and past your head causing you to overbalance. You can correct this in the same way as before, by pushing down hard with your fingertips.

3. Hold the handstand for as long as possible and then perform a controlled descent.

As one of the harder movements this is really verging on advanced calisthenics so don't be disheartened if it takes a while to learn. Just use the knowledge you already have about correcting under / over balance and with time you will nail it!

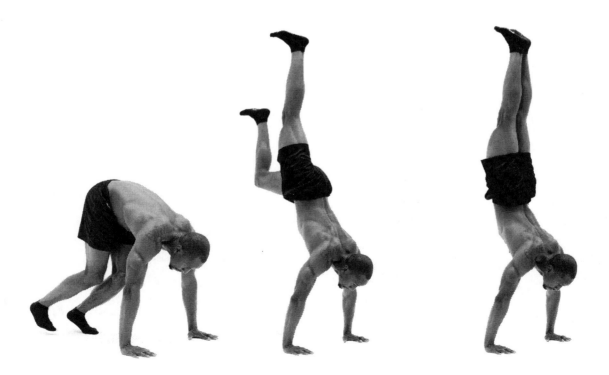

WALL SUPPORT PARALLETTE HANDSTAND

When we think of calisthenics, we often think of people upside-down on parallettes. Here's step one to mastering this coveted exercise.

Perform: maximum hold time possible.

You will need: parallettes, a sturdy wall.

1. Push the parallettes up against the wall a bit wider than shoulder width apart.

2. Gripping the parallettes firmly in the middle, push off with one leg and swing the other over until both come up against the wall, just as you did when learning the free handstand.

3. Hold for as long as you can, then reverse the movement to come down.

Remember to practice bringing your legs off the wall to get used to the free position.

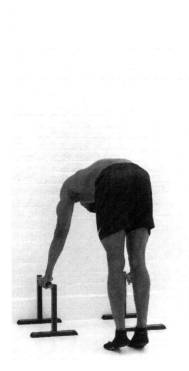
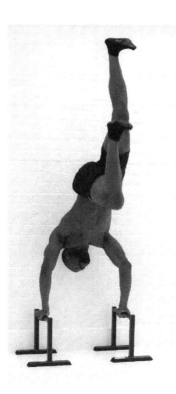
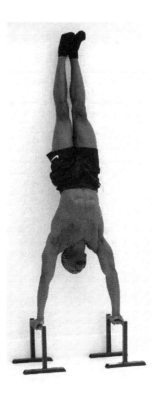

PARALLETTE HANDSTAND

Here it is, one of the most popular exercises in the calisthenics community. Prepare to test every sinew of your body to the max, with the added ingredient of superhuman stability. This is the kind of strength one can only acquire through bodyweight exercise!

Super important: Make sure you have mastered the bailout before attempting this, or any other handstand, and always give yourself ample recovery time afterwards.

Perform: maximum hold time possible.

You will need: parallettes.

1. Grip the Parallettes about shoulder width apart.

2. Bend down and push up into a handstand. As your legs swing over, push on the bars to prevent your momentum from carrying your legs too far.

3. Keep your core engaged and hold for as long as possible, remembering the stability techniques you have learned to combat under / overbalance.

NB: You can bail out of this exercise with the same style of 'cartwheel' movement we've covered before.

The straighter you keep your arms when doing this, the further your head will be from the ground, which is a good thing.

Don't lock up and grip the parallettes hard, otherwise they will come over with you. Instead, get used to pivoting and releasing.

This exercise takes guts, determination, brute strength and a whole lot of practice. It is where men become men, and boys quit and remain boys. If you make it to perfect form then you are one of the elite few, so be sure to celebrate your achievement!

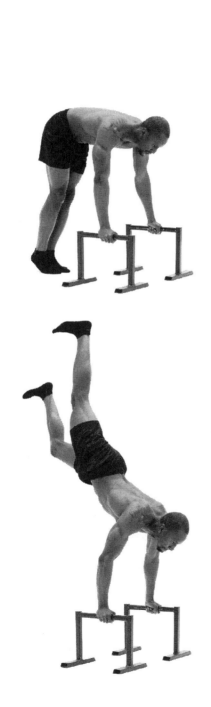
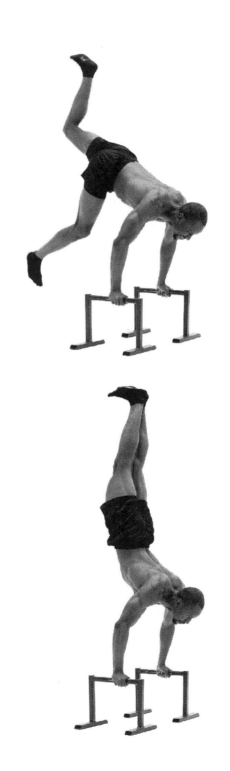

WALL SUPPORT HANDSTAND PUSH-UP

This is the first step for handstand push-ups. You'll be using the wall as a brace for your feet; therefore, you can focus on your push-up form and strength. Balance without the wall will come next. It's a good idea to use a spotter when starting out with this.

Perform: 3-4 sets of 3-5 reps.

You will need: a sturdy wall.

1. Place your hands about one foot from the wall, shoulder width apart.

2. Kick up into a wall handstand as you've already learnt.

3. Begin to lower yourself straight down by bending your elbows. Be careful not to come down hard and bang your head. A folded towel makes a great buffer.

4. When your head is nearly touching the ground, push yourself back up to the handstand position with locked out arms to complete a rep.

As before, you can practice coming away from the wall gradually before going for the full version of this exercise.

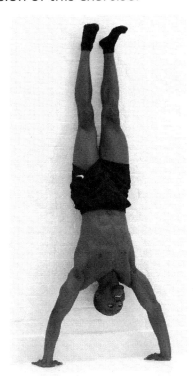 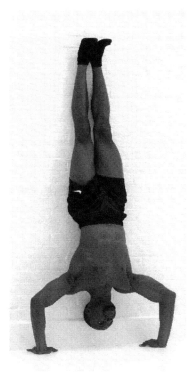

FLOOR / FREE HANDSTAND PUSH-UP

Once your strength and form have developed from the wall assisted handstand push-ups, it's time to move away from the wall. We'll be targeting your balance with this variation; remember to engage your core to center your body, and don't expect to jump straight into the same amount of reps you can perform on the wall!

Perform: 3-4 sets of 3-5 reps.

1. Pick an open spot on the floor, and place your hands about shoulder width apart.

2. Give a good kick, and launch into a handstand. Try out different positions with your legs until you find that combination that helps with your balance.

3. Once you have control, and your arms are fully extended, begin to lower yourself by bending at the elbows.

4. When your head is nearly touching the floor, push down firmly and raise yourself back up to your starting position to complete 1 rep.

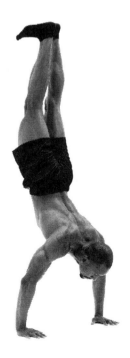
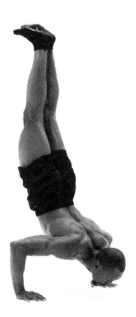

WALL SUPPORT PARALLETTE HANDSTAND PUSH-UP

To continue building on the strength developed in the previous handstand push-up variations, throw some parallettes into the mix. These will allow you to lower yourself further and increase the range of motion for the movement. For this particular version, we'll move back to the wall for a little support.

Perform: 3-4 sets of 3-5 reps.

You will need: a sturdy wall and parallettes.

1. Place the parallettes on the floor about shoulder width apart, and position them so that your hands will be about a foot from the base of the wall.

2. Grasp the parallettes and raise yourself up into the handstand position as you have already learnt, using the wall as a stop for your feet.

3. Once you are in control, arms locked out, begin to lower yourself by bending at the elbows. Remember to use a spotter and a buffer between your head and the ground at first.

4. Once your head is almost touching the floor, reverse the movement and push yourself back up to the starting position. Remember to keep your core tight and use the wall for support. That is 1 rep done!

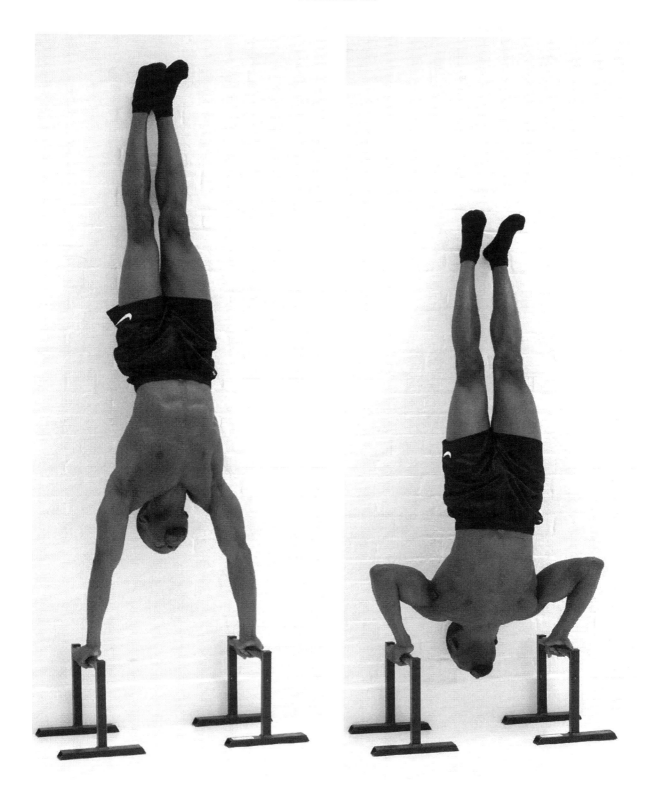

PARALLETTE HANDSTAND PUSH-UP

Once you are comfortable with the strength and range of motion required to perform the parallette handstand push-up on the wall, it is once again time to move away from additional support. This variation will challenge you to your maintain balance while at the same time exerting the strength required to complete the movement.

Perform: 3-4 sets of 2-5 reps.

You will need: parallettes.

1. Place the parallettes about shoulder width apart and grasp them firmly.

2. Raise yourself up into the handstand position, making sure to maintain tension throughout your body.

3. Once you are completely vertical, with arms locked out and in control, begin to lower yourself by bending at the elbows.

4. When your head is nearly touching the floor, push hard onto the parallettes and raise yourself back to the starting position. Congrats, that's 1 rep!

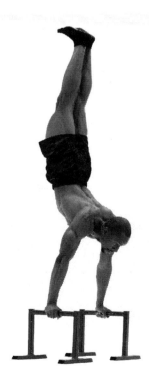

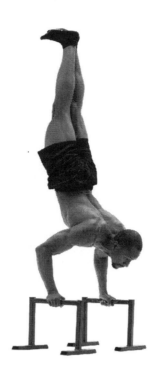

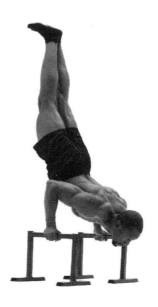

90-DEGREE PUSH-UP

As we continue to progress through the handstand push-up variations, this last exercise combines all the strength and technique we have accumulated thus far.

This is another exercise for which we advise having some kind of support structure in place. A matted area will prevent hard falls, while a spotter can provide stability and reassurance where needed.

Needless to say, this movement is incredibly taxing. Use slow, controlled, movements, add in a heavy helping of patience, and you will succeed!

Perform: 2-3 sets of 2-3 reps.

1. Place your hands about shoulder width apart, and raise yourself into the standard handstand position.

2. Once you have control, and your arms are locked out, begin to lower yourself as you would for a handstand push-up.

3. As your body is lowering, allow your shoulders to shift in front of your hands and your lower body to begin to take a horizontal orientation.

4. At the bottom of the motion, your body should be completely parallel with the ground, elbows bent at about 90°.

5. From this bottom position, push down hard and engage your core, raising your feet to reverse the motion and get yourself back to the start point. That is 1 rep of arguably the toughest push-up in the world!

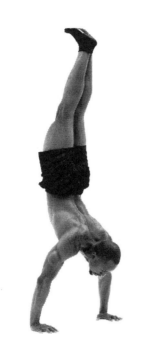

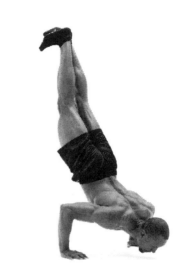

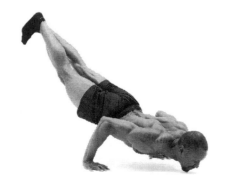

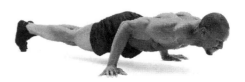

UPPER BODY LEVERS

After all you've been through you would be forgiven for thinking you have 'completed' calisthenics. However, we're just getting started! So far we've largely been in motion, and it's now time to delve into isometric - or static - exercises. This is where calisthenics comes into its own. Prepare to level up, comrade. The road to SUPERHUMAN continues!

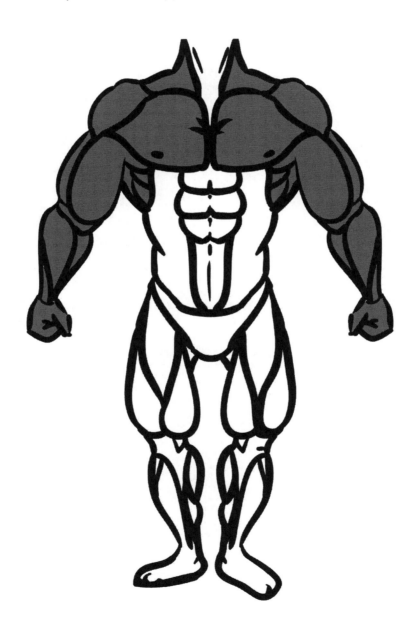

FRONT LEVER

The front lever is extremely difficult, so we'll take it in manageable steps, working to slowly move your legs away from your core and extend them all the way out. Repetition is key here. Keep holding position for as long as you can and you will achieve mastery.

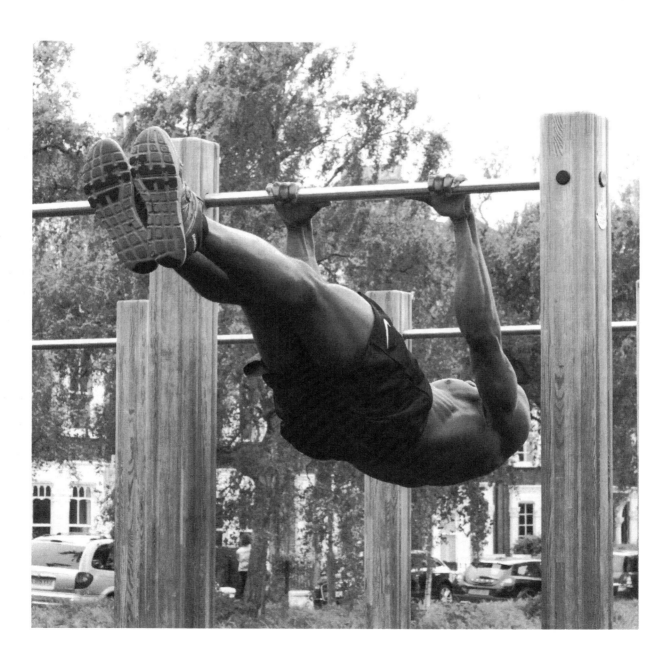

STRAIGHT PULL

As we branch into the field of the front lever, it's important to develop the concept of pulling down on the bar without bending at the elbows. To practice this skill, work on this straightforward vertical pull maneuver.

Perform: 10-20 second hold time.

You will need: pull-up bar.

1. Assume the standard pull-up position by grasping the bar with an overhand grip and keeping your hands shoulder width apart.

2. Begin from a dead hang, with arms completely locked out. Now pull your shoulders away and down from your ears. Remember to keep your arms straight!

3. Now begin to lean back a little while pulling hard on the bar. Try to close the angle between your arms and chest. As you get stronger, the gap will close further and further until you are able to get closer to the full front lever.

4. Hold for as long as possible, then drop off the bar and reset.

NB: If you are going into this exercise without any prior practice on the bar, then you will likely find it impossible.

We've mentioned several times that this is a progressive calisthenics guide, so if you cannot complete this movement please go back and cover the previous exercises.

As with all foundation exercises, straight pulls will take great patience to conquer. Once you have achieved perfect form, though, you will find the following exercises come much more naturally to you.

Front Lever

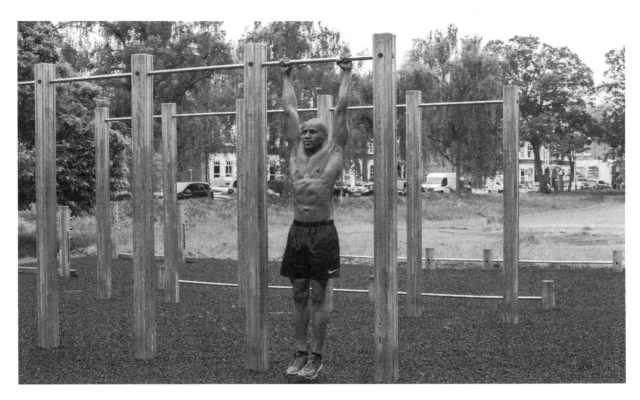

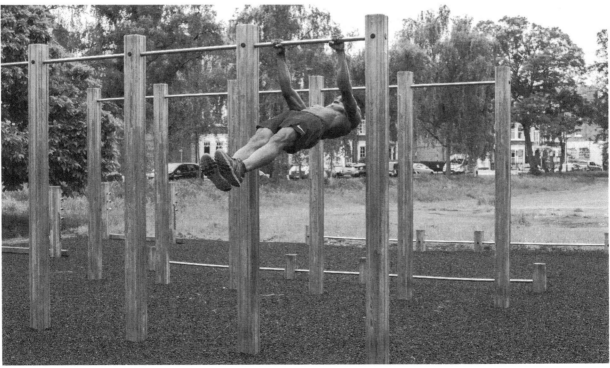

TUCK FRONT LEVER

When you've nailed the straight pull, it's time to tackle the front tuck front lever. We'll begin to engage the core with this position, keeping your legs close and tucked up to your chest to limit the strain to begin with.

Perform: 10-20 second hold time.

You will need: pull-up bar.

1. Assume the standard pull-up position, and allow yourself to hang with your arms completely locked out.

2. Engage your core, and pull your knees up to your chest. You should pivot so that your back is facing the ground.

3. Continue to pull down on the bar with your arms locked out, and hold for as long as possible. When you feel strong enough to up your game, let your knees come away from your chest so your hips align with your shoulders, achieving a straight back.

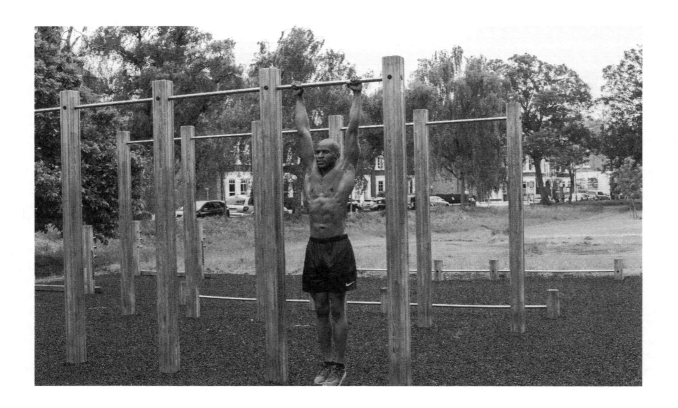

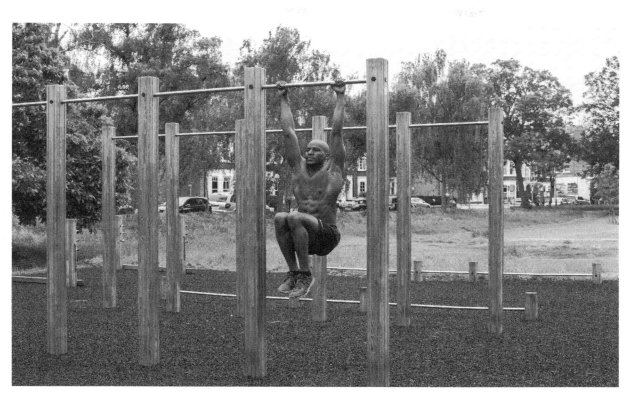

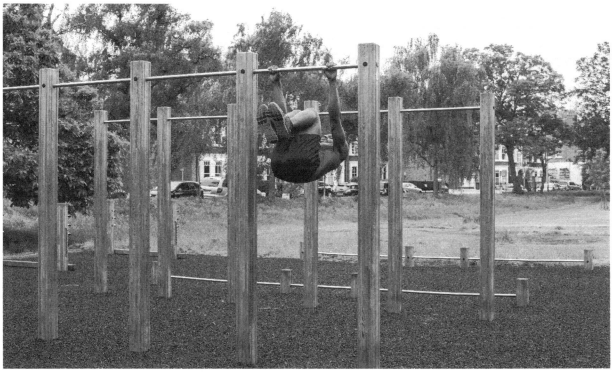

SINGLE-LEG FRONT LEVER

Mastered the tuck position for the specified length of time? Then we can proceed to the single-leg version. Focus on maintaining rigidity throughout your extended leg and keeping it straight for the entire duration.

Perform: 10-20 second hold time.

You will need: pull-up bar.

1. Assume the tuck back lever position that we have already presented.

2. Extend one leg straight out while keeping the other tucked up to your chest. Point your toe in the extended leg to help maintain rigidity.

3. Hold for as long as possible, then switch legs.

NB: You might go into variations like this thinking that something as simple as sticking a leg out will be a simple variation on an exercise you have already mastered.

Well, hold the champagne for now, because calisthenics doesn't quite work like that! You will quickly discover that even the subtlest variations can call to action completely different parts of your body which have not been used before.

This can be an incredibly frustrating experience, but you mustn't be disheartened. If you've made it this far then you have already proven that progress is possible.

Keep training one step at a time, and be sure to keep a training journal so that you have something to look back on and remind yourself how far you have already come.

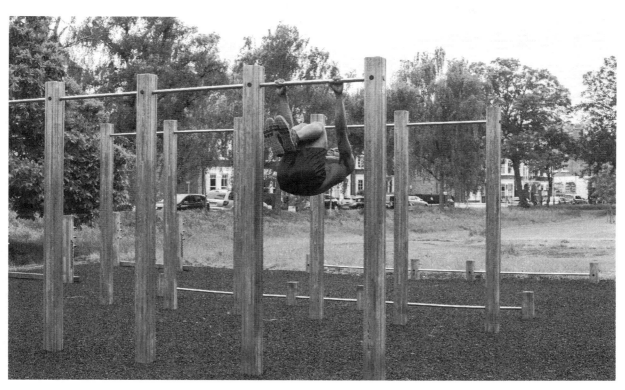

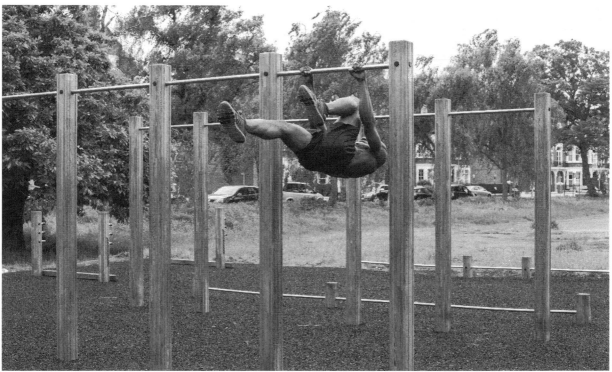

SPLAYED FRONT LEVER FROM TOP SWING

Next up we need to learn the splayed front lever. We'll start by using momentum, swinging your body down from a pull-up or muscle-up position and straight into the lever. This is requires full great upper body and core control throughout the movement.

Perform: 10-15 second hold time.

You will need: pull-up bar.

1. Grasp the bar in the standard pull-up orientation, and pull your chin over the top. Experiment with heights until you find one that feels natural when going into the next movement. You may even wish to go all the way up top at first.

2. Now tighten your core and lower body. Begin to lower yourself from the top, and swing your lower body forward and under the bar at the same time. Think of 'sliding' down into the splayed lever.

3. At the bottom, your legs should be out in front of you in a wide 'V' position, your arms will be locked out, and your shoulders level with your feet.

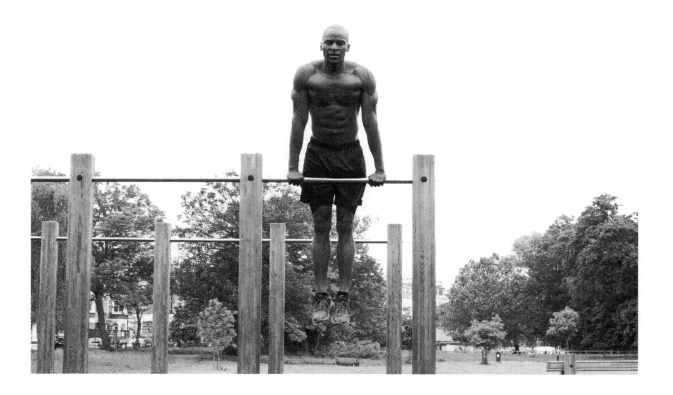

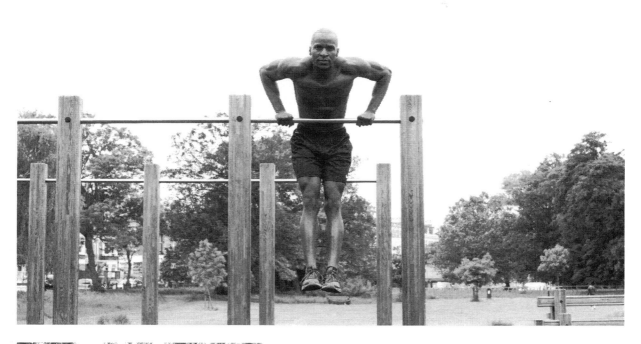

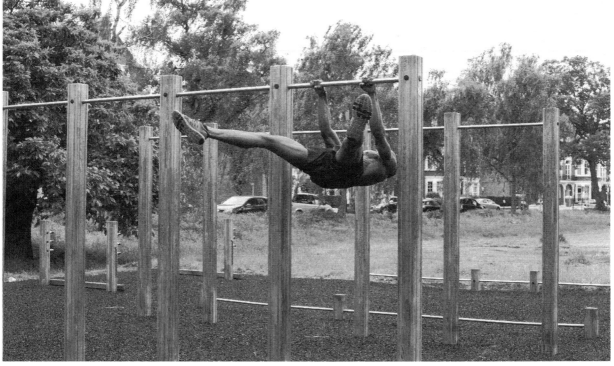

Splayed Front Lever from Bottom Swing

This is another great hack for getting into the splayed front lever, starting from a dead hang and using a well-known exercise to get you there.

Perform: 10-15 second hold time.

You will need: pull-up bar.

1. Grasp the bar in the standard pull-up orientation, and perform a leg raise from a dead hang.

2. In a controlled movement, lower your legs down and open them out gradually.

3. At the bottom, your legs should be out in front of you in a wide 'V' position, your arms will be locked out, and your shoulders level with your feet.

NB: The first step in this exercise is also known as a leg raise. We'll cover that in core exercises later, so don't worry if you don't quite possess the leg strength or flexibility to pull it off just yet - there is always a way to build up to it!

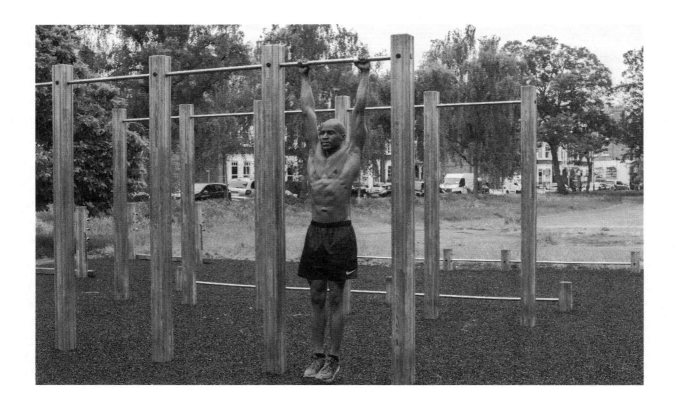

Front Lever

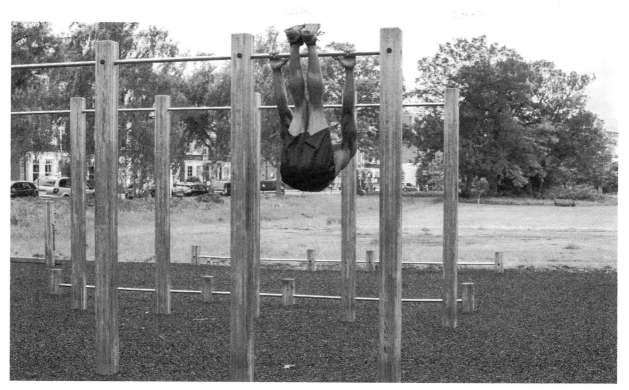

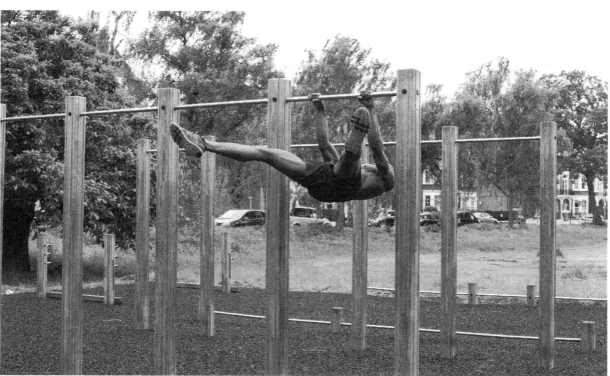

SPLAYED FRONT LEVER FROM TUCK

This is another method to get yourself into the splayed front lever, which will require a great deal of core strength and control, but will therefore yield great benefit to your overall strength.

Perform: 10-15 second hold time.

You will need: pull-up bar.

1. Assume the front tuck lever position that was covered earlier.

2. Slowly extend both legs out into a 'V' shape. Remember to control your breathing as you complete this motion, and maintain control.

3. Once both legs are fully extended, and your body is straight from head to toe, hold for as long as possible.

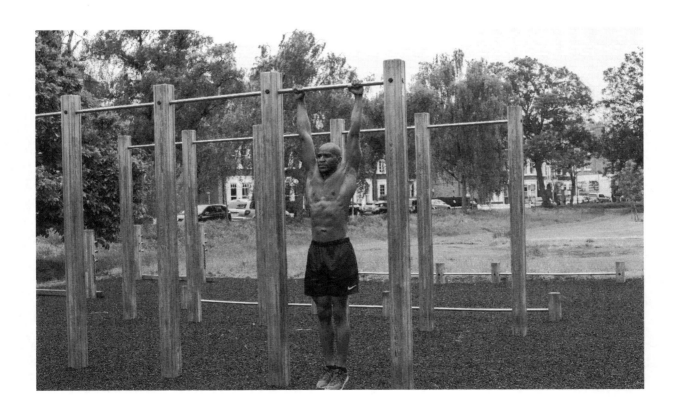

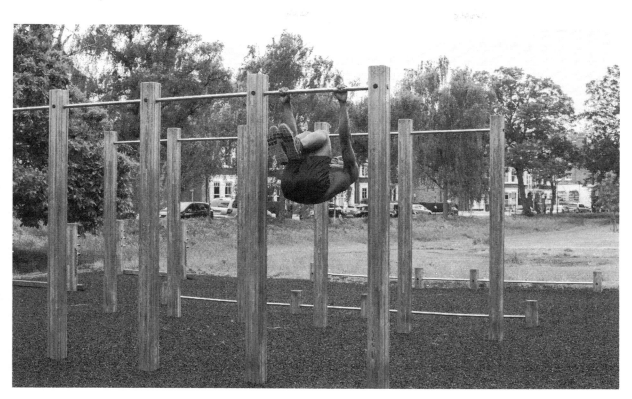

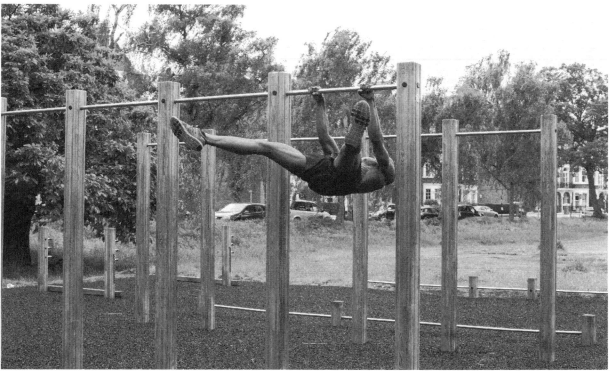

COMPLETE FRONT LEVER

The front lever is not fully mastered until you bring your legs together. Although only a minor change from the splayed position, this will tax your core to the extreme, and will take a great deal of practice to maintain.

Perform: 10-15 second hold time.

You will need: pull-up bar.

1. Assume the splayed or tuck front lever using the methods described previously.

2. Bring your legs together from splayed position, closing the 'V', or extend them straight out from tuck, and hold for as long as possible.

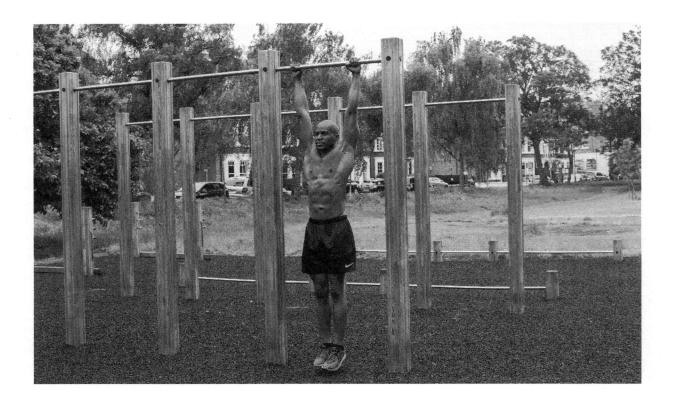

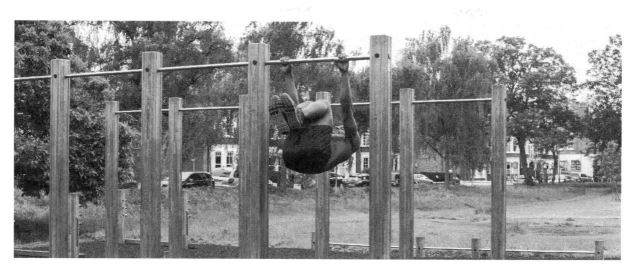

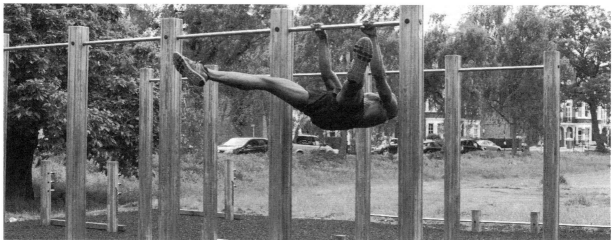

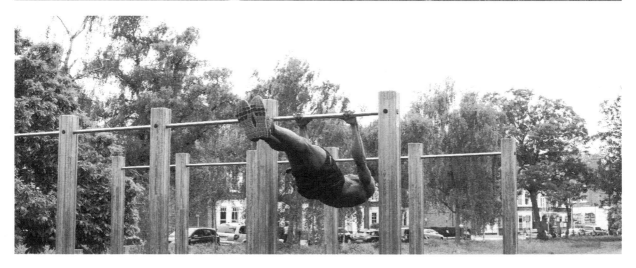

FRONT LEVER PULL-UPS

Still not tough enough for you? Then toss in some pull-ups! This variation combines all the standard aspects of the front lever, but includes pull-ups for an additional challenge.

NB: When starting out it is a good idea to begin practicing these in the tucked position as shown. Once mastered, move onto splayed and then the complete version for a more intense workout.

Since you have already seen all the available variations, simply apply them to whichever front lever pull-up you wish to perform.

Perform: 3-4 sets of 3-5 reps.

You will need: pull-up bar.

1. Assume the front lever position of your choice, as presented before.

2. Once in position, begin to pull yourself up to the bar while maintaining the position, aiming to get your chest as close to the metal as possible.

3. When you reach the top, slowly lower yourself back to the starting position while maintaining tension throughout your body. That's a rep!

That concludes this collection of front lever exercises. If you've managed to master this complex movement then you have our express permission to pat yourself on the back.

Remember to go back and brush up on the foundation exercises if you still need to work on certain aspects. Most advanced calisthenics movements take years to truly master, so be sure to keep this guide handy!

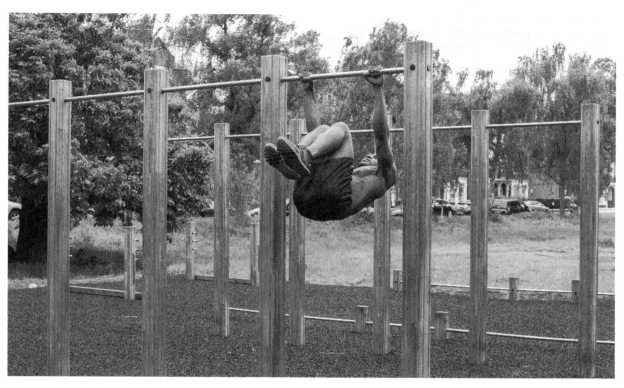

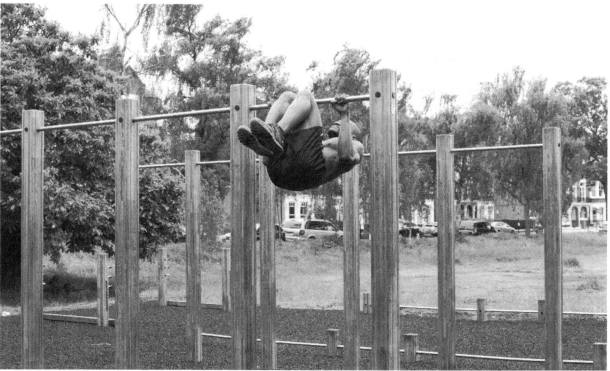

BACK LEVER

It's now time to take on the back lever. This will put massive strain on your shoulders so ensure that you complete your warm-ups before jumping in. We'll follow a very similar progression to the front lever, starting with the essential foundation exercises. Let's go!

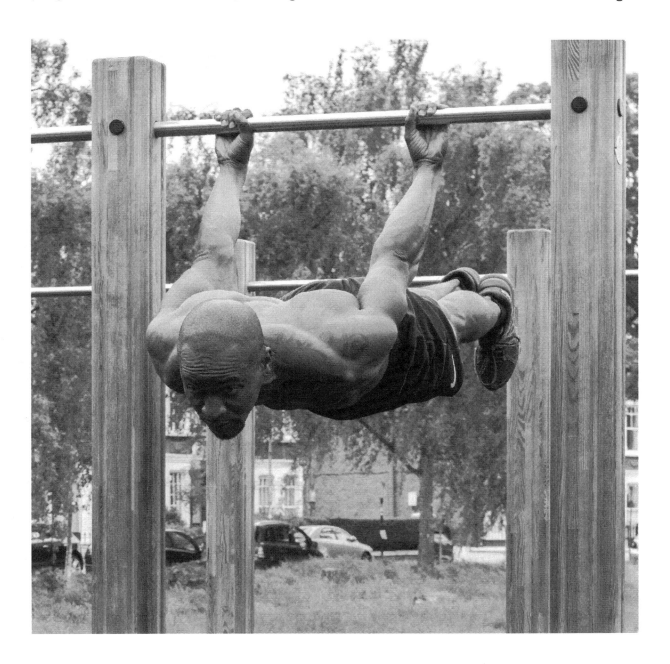

SKIN THE CAT

Before we begin to challenge the core in the back lever positions, we'll first focus on your shoulder mobility and strength. This position will feel uncomfortable and unstable to start with, so take it slow and concentrate on increasing your range of motion.

Perform: 10-15 second hold time.

You will need: pull-up bar.

1. Grasp the bar in the standard pull-up position with locked out arms and an overhand grip.

2. Now engage your core and bring your legs up in a leg raise, while at the same time leaning backwards.

3. Bend your knees enough to bring your legs all the way through the gap between your arms, continuing your backward momentum.

4. Carry on rotating until you are facing forwards once more, with your legs hanging underneath you, and hold for as long as possible

Remember: This book is designed to teach calisthenics in a progressive manner. If you're finding something too difficult, don't try to 'power through.'

If you are truly committed to calisthenics then you must understand that it is a gradual learning curve. Take a step back, assess your progress and, if necessary, revisit earlier exercises to work on your foundational strength.

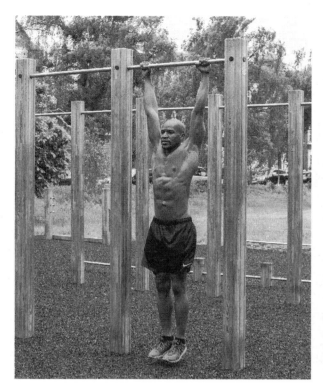
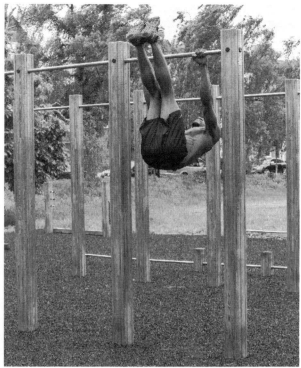
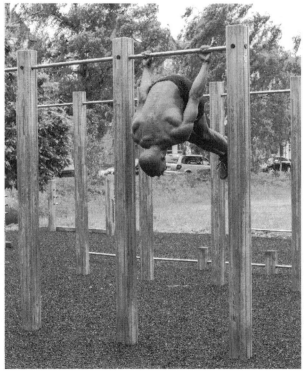
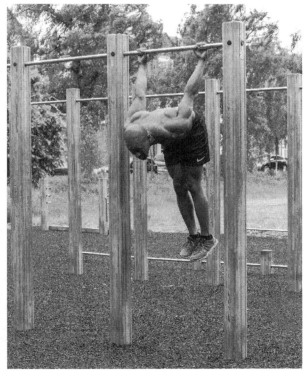

TUCK BACK LEVER

Once you are comfortable holding the previous position for the time specified, then we can begin to add complexity and make the position more difficult. We'll start with the tuck back lever which will simply involve bringing your knees up.

OK, we say 'simply', but we all know by now that making the next step in any variation or progression can be maddeningly difficult.

There is no shame in using a spotter to help you get in position or take some of the strain away from the hold. What's important is that once you become comfortable with that, you begin to practice under your own steam.

Perform: 10-15 second hold time.

You will need: pull-up bar.

1. Assume the 'skin the cat' position as previously covered.

2. Bring your knees up as close to your chest as possible, while raising your hips to about the same height as your shoulders.

3. Hold for as long as possible.

Remember: If you can't hit the allotted hold time for this exercise, break it down into chunks. For example, 2 x 5 seconds or 3 x 5 seconds.

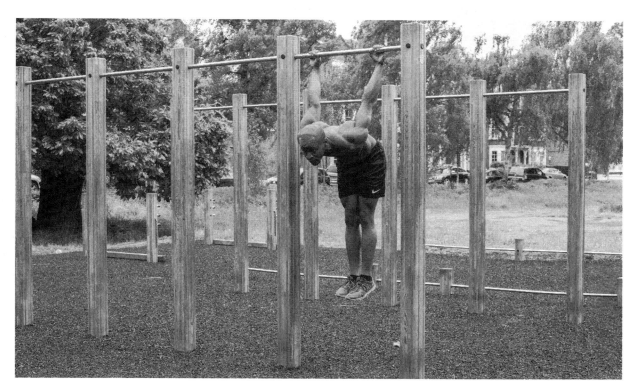

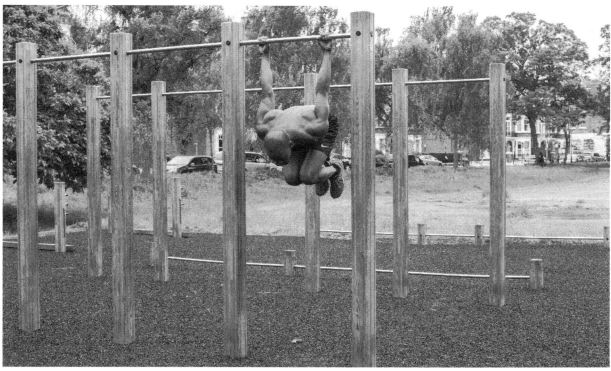

SINGLE-LEG BACK LEVER

As you probably expected, once you can maintain the tuck back lever, it's time to bring those legs out! We'll start with one leg in order to develop the immense core strength and stability required to hold it.

Perform: 10-20 second hold time.

You will need: pull-up bar.

1. Assume the tuck back lever position from the previous exercise.

2. Extend one leg straight out behind you while keeping the other tucked up. Breathe normally and point your toes to keep your form in check.

3. Hold for as long as possible.

Remember: When working single-leg, or any one-sided movement, always perform the same exercise on the other side afterwards, otherwise you run the risk of developing a muscular imbalance.

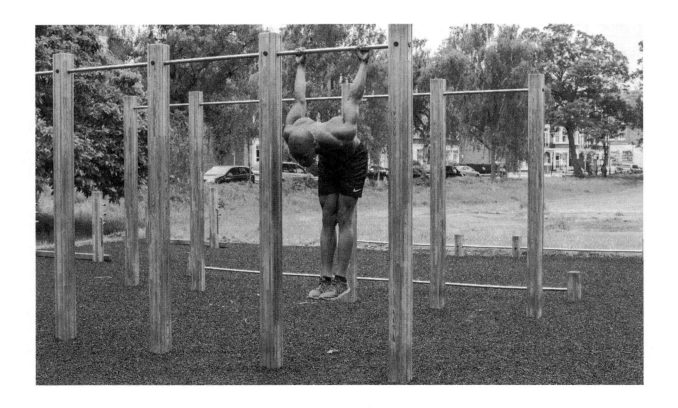

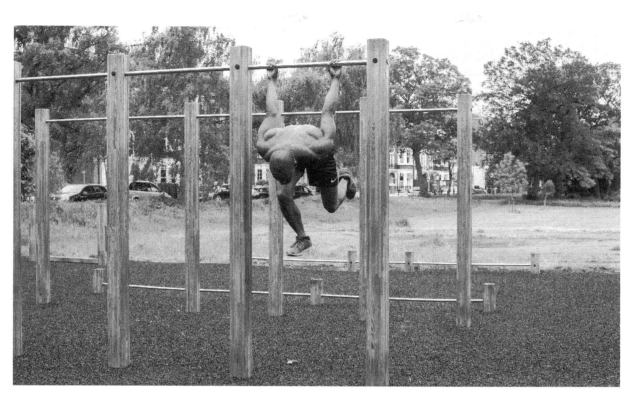

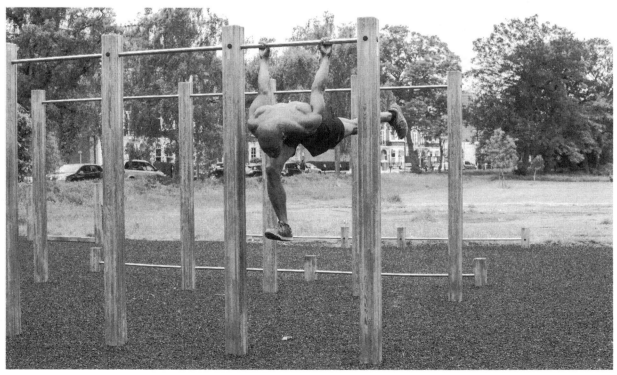

SPLAYED BACK LEVER

When you can hold a single leg back lever for the time specified, move on to extending both legs out behind you in the splayed back lever. This greatly increases the strain on your shoulders and core, so take it slow!

Perform: 10-20 second hold time.

You will need: pull-up bar.

1. Assume the tuck back lever position.

2. Slowly extend both legs out behind you in a wide 'V' formation.

3. Hold for as long as possible.

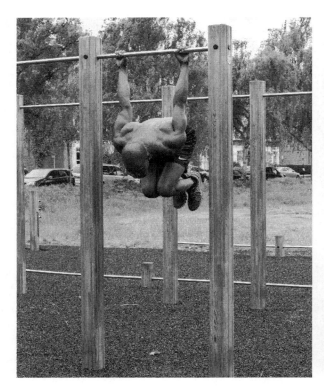
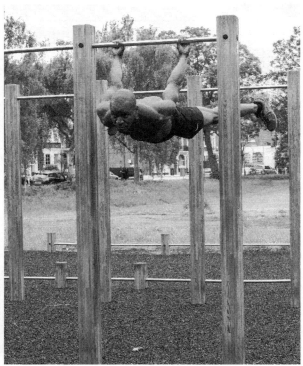

COMPLETE BACK LEVER

Bringing both legs together for the full back lever will push your core and shoulders even further. At first, you may only be able to hold this position for a second or two, but keep at it.

Perform: 10-20 second hold time.

You will need: pull-up bar.

1. Assume the splayed or tuck back lever as presented previously.

2. Now bring your legs together to eliminate the 'V' from splayed, or stick them straight out from tucked. Remember to point your toes to help stay rigid.

3. Hold for as long as possible, then drop off the bar and celebrate! That's back levers all wrapped up.

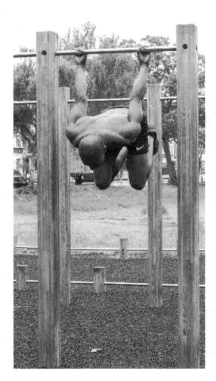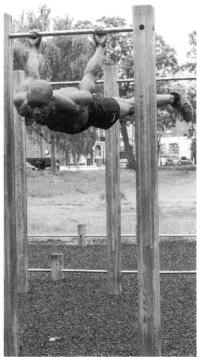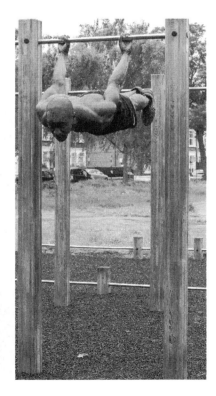

PLANCHE

Prepare to put your upper body through hell in the name of SERIOUS gains! If you're ready to defy gravity and take another step towards SUPERHUMAN then start here, and remember to master the fundamental foundation exercises before trying the real thing.

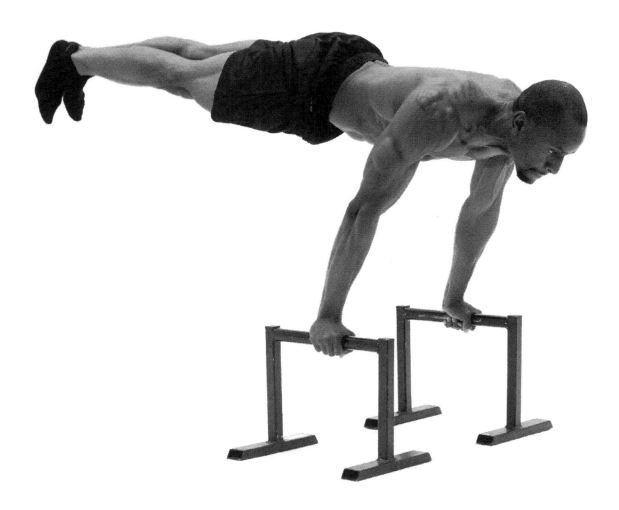

PLANCHE LEAN

This simple pose is your starting point for building the upper body strength and stability required to pull off the big one later down the line.

Perform: 3-4 sets of 10-20 second holds.

1. Get into regular push-up position with your elbows locked.

2. Slowly walk your feet forward, keeping your hands rooted, so that your shoulders move past and in front of your hands.

3. Stretch out your scapulae as if you were trying to get your shoulders to touch in front of you and raise your spine as high as possible.

4. Once you are at maximum stretch, hold to complete one set.

Variation: Use parallettes instead of the floor.

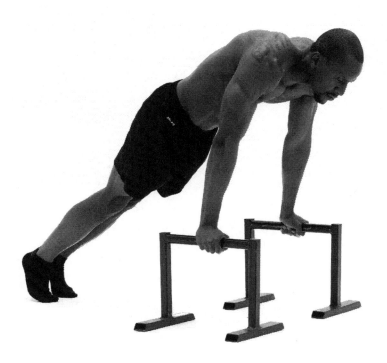

FROG STAND

The next progression in the lever exercise group is the frog stand, which helps condition your hands, wrists and arms and upper body in preparation for further progress.

Perform: 10-20 second hold time.

1. Place your hands flat on the floor in front of you, fingers facing forward in the most natural position for you.

2. Crouching down like a frog, bring your knees forward and rest them against the outsides of your elbows.

3. Push down hard with your hands and slowly let your feet lift off the floor, leaning forward slightly if it helps your balance.

4. Hold this position until you reach the allotted time. If you can't complete the allotted time, perform as many sets as it takes to do e.g. 2 x 10 seconds.

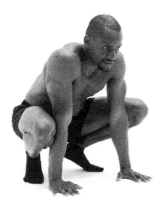
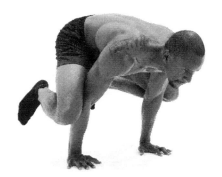

TUCK PLANCHE

This exercise preps you for all other forms of the planche to come later down the line.

Perform: 10-20 second hold time.

You will need: parallettes if you wish.

1. Place your hands on the parallettes and lift your feet off the ground.

2. Bring your knees up towards your chest, supporting your bodyweight on your wrists.

3. Lean forward until your upper bodyweight counterbalances your lower bodyweight and try to hold this position. Once again, perform as many sets as it takes to hit your allotted time.

Variations:

• Ditch the parallettes and go on the floor!

• You can also perform the exercise with your fingers pointing backwards to engage your biceps more if doing this on the floor.

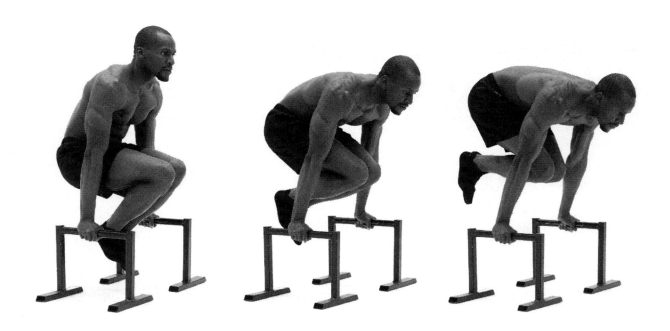

STRAIGHT BACK PLANCHE

When you can hold the tuck planche for approximately 30 seconds, you can graduate to the flat back variation. The subtle but crucial difference being that we will now maintain a completely flat back during the hold, which will engage your core and shoulders.

Perform: 10-20 second hold time.

1. Place your hands on the ground approx shoulder width apart, and raise yourself into the tuck planche position.

2. Once there, continue to raise your hips until they are at about the same level as your shoulders, so your back should be straight.

3. Engage your core and lock out your arms, and maintain for allotted time.

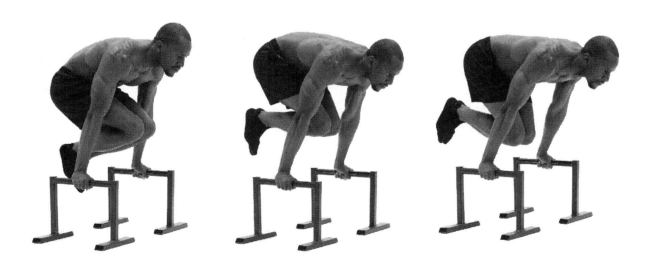

SINGLE-LEG PLANCHE

Continuing our planche progression, once you have mastered the flat back planche then it's time to move on to the single-leg variation.

This requires you to hold one leg out behind you while keeping the other tucked up to your torso. Sound familiar?

As you will know by now, we're working towards eventually having both legs stretched out behind, so focus on your breathing, balance, and control as we move forward.

Perform: 10-20 second hold time.

You will need: parallettes if you wish.

1. Assume the straight back planche position described previously, ensuring you have total control of your body before moving onto the next step.

2. Once your back is straight, extend one leg out behind you while keeping the other tucked up.

3. Maintain this position for the allotted time, aiming to keep the line between your foot, hips and shoulders as straight as possible.

Variation: Switch legs without coming down if you want to turn this into a sets and reps style exercise. This will also bring your core into the equation much more than it already is, so you can even revisit this when training for that popping six-pack later on!

NB: Those training without parallettes might find this more difficult. For a stronger grip and greater ground clearance, consider using parallettes, at least when getting started.

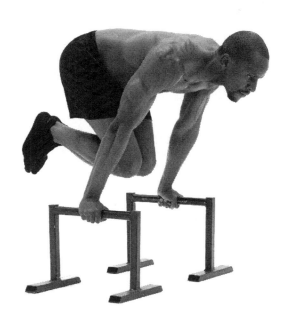

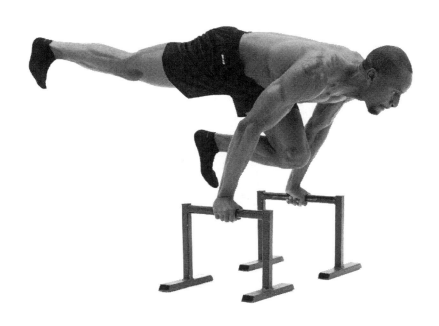

SPLAYED PLANCHE FROM SWING

Continuing along a familiar path, we're now going to use the swing method as a break-in for the proper splayed planche. In this case, we'll be using parallettes and gentle momentum to achieve the desired outcome.

Perform: 10-20 second hold time.

You will need: parallettes.

1. Grasp the parallettes and assume a half lever (also known as an L sit) or tuck half lever (knees drawn in).

2. Swing your legs back through your arms and lean forward slightly, using the gentle momentum to carry you through, opening your legs out wide as you go.

3. Once you're in the splayed planche, hold for as long as possible.

Variation: Reverse and repeat to turn this into a sets and reps style exercise.

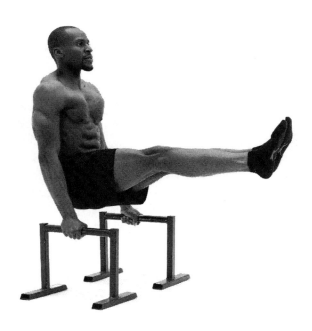

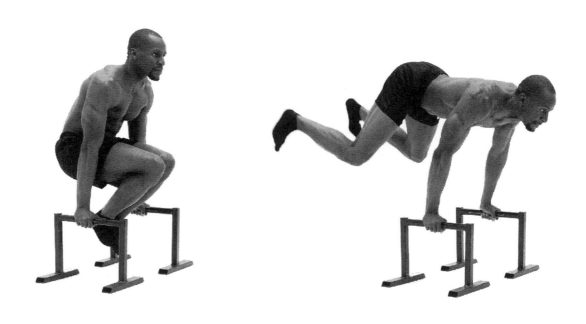

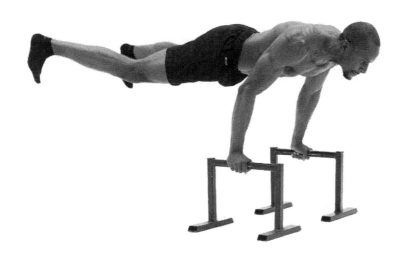

SPLAYED PLANCHE FROM TUCK

Here's another way to get into the splayed planche, this time starting from the tuck planche that you have already learnt.

Perform: 10-20 second hold time.

You will need: parallettes if you wish.

1. Assume the tuck planche position that we have already covered.

2. Now extend both of them out behind you in a 'V' shape. The wider the V, the easier it will be to hold the position.

3. Maintain your breathing, and hold your entire body as straight as you can for the allotted time.

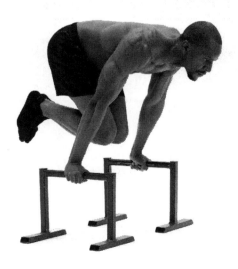

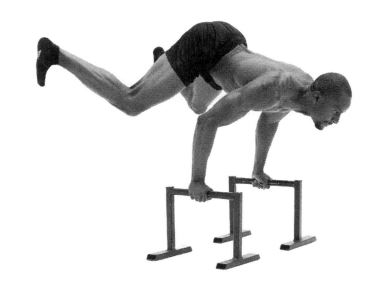

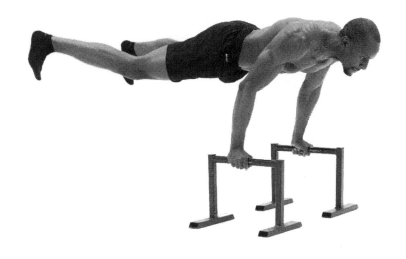

SPLAYED PLANCHE FROM PULL

Here we will cover how to transition from a push-up style position all the way to the splayed planche. This movement will require you to contract your core and back as hard as you possibly can to maintain a flat posture as you lift off the ground.

Perform: 10-20 second hold time.

You will need: parallettes if you wish.

1. Assume a planche lean style position with your hands on the parallettes, shoulder width apart. Start with your legs in a wide 'V' position.

2. Keeping your body straight and rigid, begin to lean forward and use your hands as a pivot point to lift your legs off the ground as you transition forward.

3. Once your entire body is off the ground and rigid in the splayed planche, hold for as long as you can.

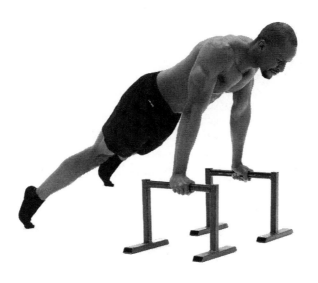

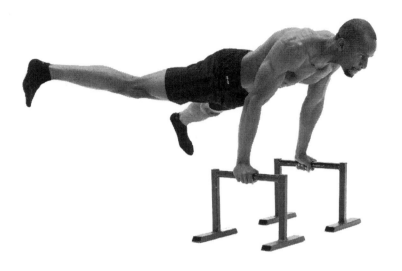

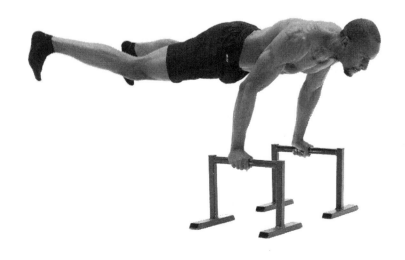

SPLAYED PLANCHE FROM HANDSTAND

While extremely difficult to master, this method of assuming the straddle planche will immeasurably increase your strength and balance. Remember to take it slow, and one step at a time!

Perform: 10-20 second hold time.

You will need: parallettes if you wish.

1. Kick up into a handstand, without wall support. Position your legs in a wide 'V'.

2. While maintaining straight arms, slowly move your shoulders forward while lowering your legs behind you. Keep your back straight!

3. Once your body is horizontal, you have reached the splayed planche position. Hold for as long as you can, and don't forget to breathe steadily.

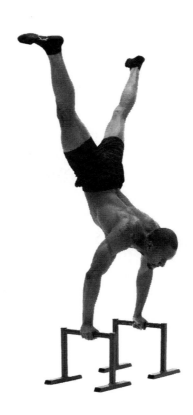

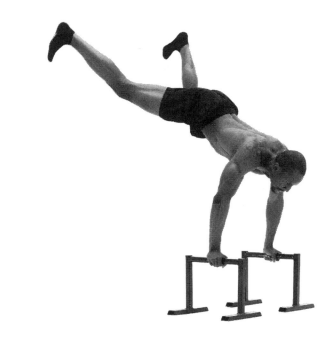

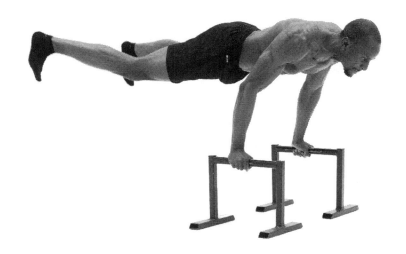

COMPLETE PLANCHE

The challenge isn't over yet! The complete planche is, in essence the same as the splayed planche, but you'll be bringing your legs together.

If you've been through similar exercise progressions before then you will know that this requires even greater core and arm strength to maintain.

Perform: 5-10 second hold time.

You will need: parallettes if you wish.

1. Assume the splayed planche position using any of the methods we have covered. We are starting from tuck in the pictures.

2. Once you are in the splayed planche, bring your legs together so they are straight and touching. Hold for as long as you can!

Remember: Though you are training to perform these exercises under your own steam, there is no harm in having a spotter help you in the early stages. Just remember not to rely on them, as this would be counter-productive.

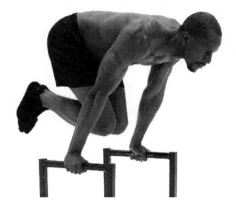

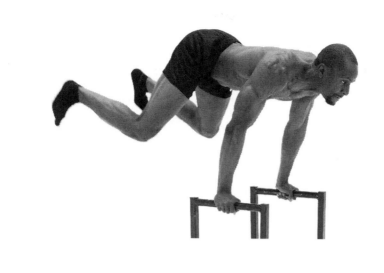

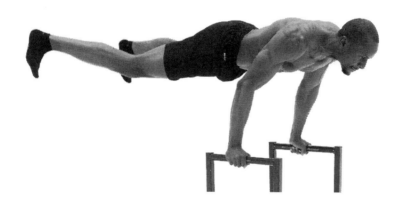

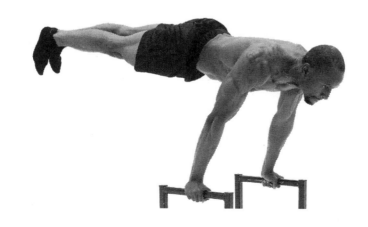

TUCK PLANCHE PUSH-UP

You are one step away from planche mastery! Before trying the full planche push-up, try this slightly easier version.

Perform: 3-4 sets of 5-8 reps.

You will need: parallettes if you wish.

1. Assume the tuck planche position using any of the techniques we have presented.

2. Bend your elbows and lower yourself down as deep as possible. You may not go far at first, but keep at it!

3. Push hard and raise yourself back up, while maintaining the planche. Your rep is complete when your arms are straight again.

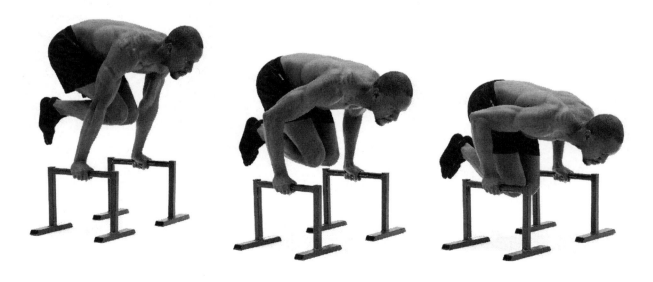

PLANCHE PUSH-UP

If you've mastered everything so far, and still aren't satisfied, we've got an upgrade for you. Try this for a serious, dynamic workout.

Perform: 3-4 sets of 3-5 reps.

You will need: parallettes if you wish.

1. Assume the planche position using any of the techniques we have presented.

2. Once you are in the planche, bend at the elbows and lower yourself until your chest is just above the floor. If on parallettes, go as deep as you can.

3. Push down hard and raise yourself back to the start, while maintaining the planche. Lock those elbows to complete 1 rep.

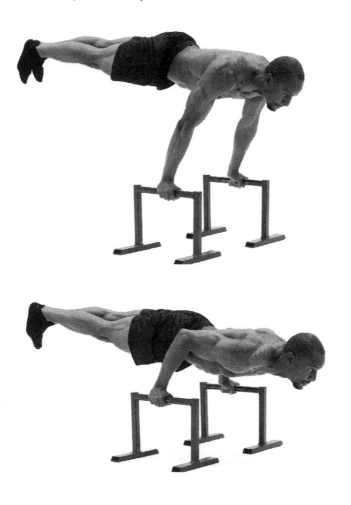

THE HUMAN FLAG

Here it is, the holy grail of all bodyweight exercises and the final frontier for achieving SUPERHUMAN upper body strength! Use the following progressive exercises to build up to the complete version. What follows will be familiar, but by no means easy. Onwards!

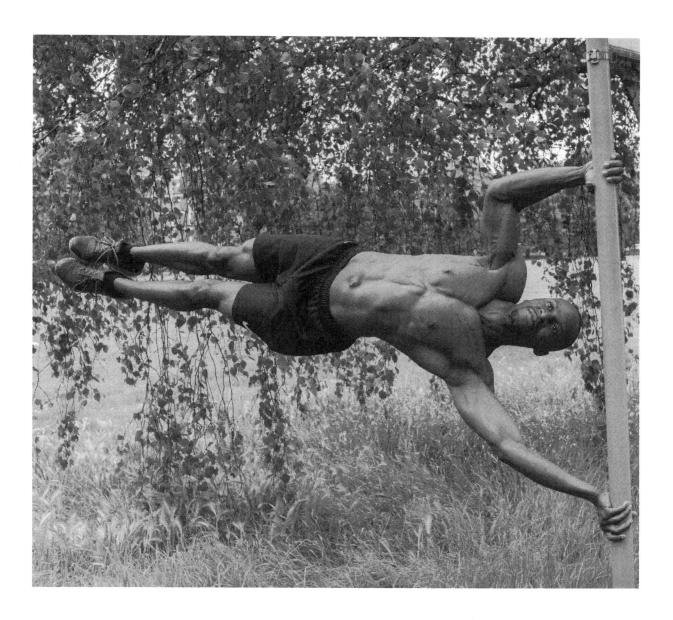

DRAPED FLAG

The first step in training for the human flag is to master the 'draped' position. This will build great strength and control, while also conditioning your body for maintaining the tension required to achieve the complete version.

Perform: 10-15 second hold time per side.

You will need: A stable, vertical pole or fixed bar.

1. Lean sideways towards the bar and grasp with your hands wide apart, the top hand using an overhand 'pulling' grip while the bottom uses an underhand 'pushing' grip.

2. Begin to pull with the arm that is placed higher on the pole, and at the same time push with the lower arm.

3. As your feet begin to leave the ground, keep your core tight and raise your feet into the air as much as you can manage. When you are first beginning this step, you may need to give yourself a little kick as you leave the ground.

4. Hold this position for allotted time.

Be sure to work both sides of your body with this exercise or you will quickly develop an imbalance. As you become more comfortable with the motion, begin to increase your hold times. Once you can hold this position steadily for more than 10 seconds you can move on to the next step.

Super important: Don't forget to check the pole or fixture you are using for this exercise is completely sturdy and can take your weight before hauling yourself into the human flag! Street signs are usually good, but only if they are well away from the roads.

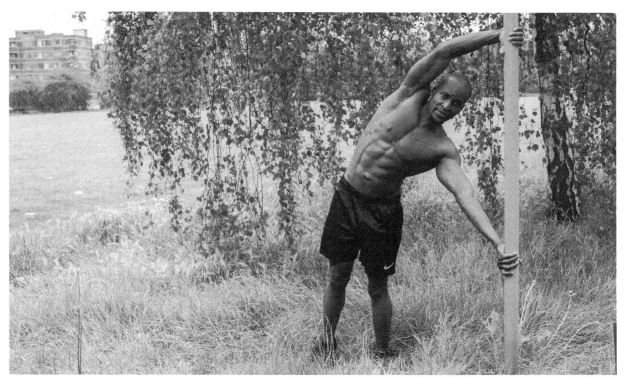

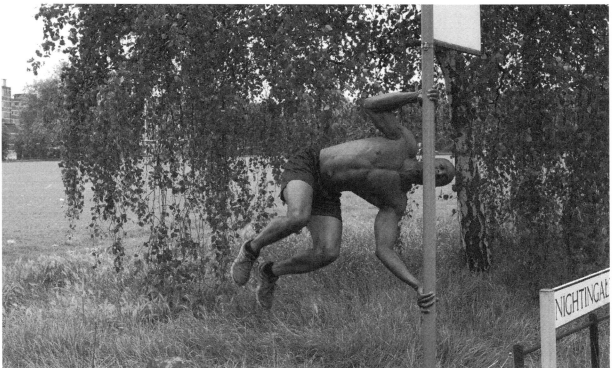

TUCKED FLAG

When your arms, shoulders and core are fully accustomed to holding the draped flag position, we can begin to neaten things up.

Perform: 10-15 second hold time per side.

You will need: stable, vertical pole or fixed bar.

1. Grasp the bar and assume the draped flag position described above. Keep your knees tucked in throughout.

2. Activate your core, lower back, and glutes, while pulling hard with your upper arm to raise yourself up further.

3. Push with your lower arm and raise your torso until it's parallel with the ground.

4. Hold for as long as possible

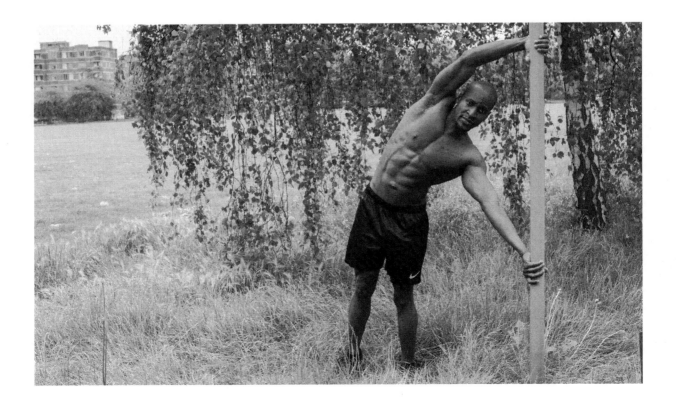

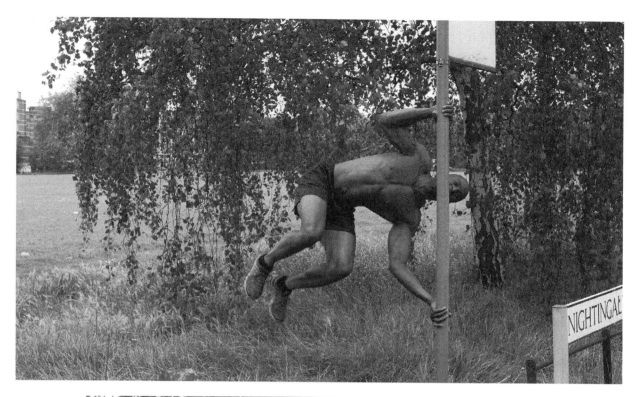

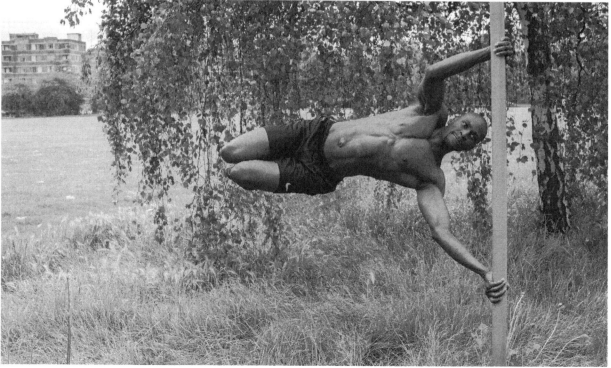

SPLAYED FLAG

You guessed it, the next step after the tucked flag is to extend those legs out and hold the splayed flag position. Remember to switch sides between sets to make sure you get an even workout.

Perform: 10-15 second hold time per side.

You will need: stable, vertical pole or fixed bar.

1. Assume the tucked flag position we established in the last exercise.

2. Now extend your legs into a wide 'V' position. If this is too difficult, experiment with different positions for your arms to see if you can get more leverage.

3. Hold for as long as possible.

Remember: The hold times suggested in this book are just a general recommendation, so they do not take into account your own personal level of ability.

As ever, if you are struggling to complete the allotted time, either take a step back to the previous exercise, or split it into a 'sets' style exercise, holding for as long as you can in each set until you reach the total allotted time.

For example, if aiming for 10 seconds, 5 x 2 second sets, or 2 x 5 second sets will help build the strength required for performing the full version.

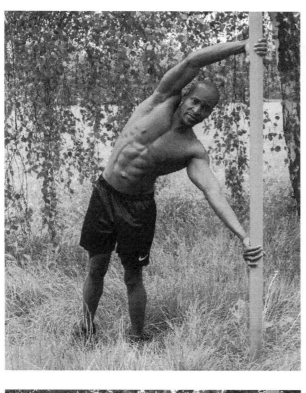
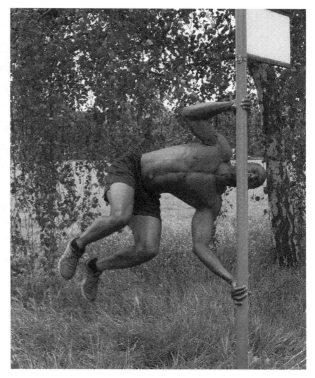
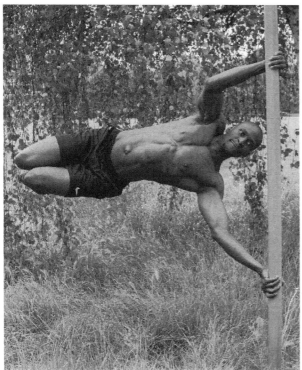
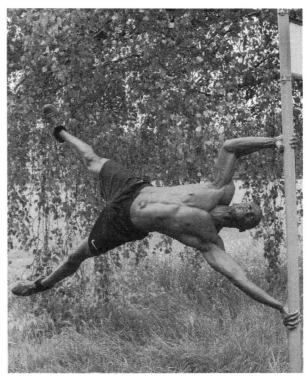

COMPLETE HUMAN FLAG

Now it's time for the big league! Once you can hold the splayed flag for the required time, bring those legs together for the full human flag and an amazing upper body and core workout.

Perform: 10-15 second hold time per side.

You will need: stable, vertical pole or fixed bar.

1. Assume the splayed flag position, or tuck flag depending on which one you are most comfortable with.

2. If coming from splayed, slowly bring your legs together until they are touching. If starting at tuck, simply extend your legs outwards (this variation is harder for most!)

3. Hold for as long as possible.

NB: This is the holy grail for us calisthenics nuts, but it is also one of the most difficult exercises in the world to perform. We've put it in the upper body section, but in truth, as with many bodyweight moves, it calls on almost every muscle group.

You will require immense upper body strength to pull off this move, as well as a super tight core and perfect lower body control.

If and when you complete this with perfect form, give yourself one huge pat on the back, because it doesn't get much tougher than this!

You are now part of the elite few who have completed Upper Body BLAST. But do not pop the champagne cork just yet, comrade, for no workout is complete without cardio!

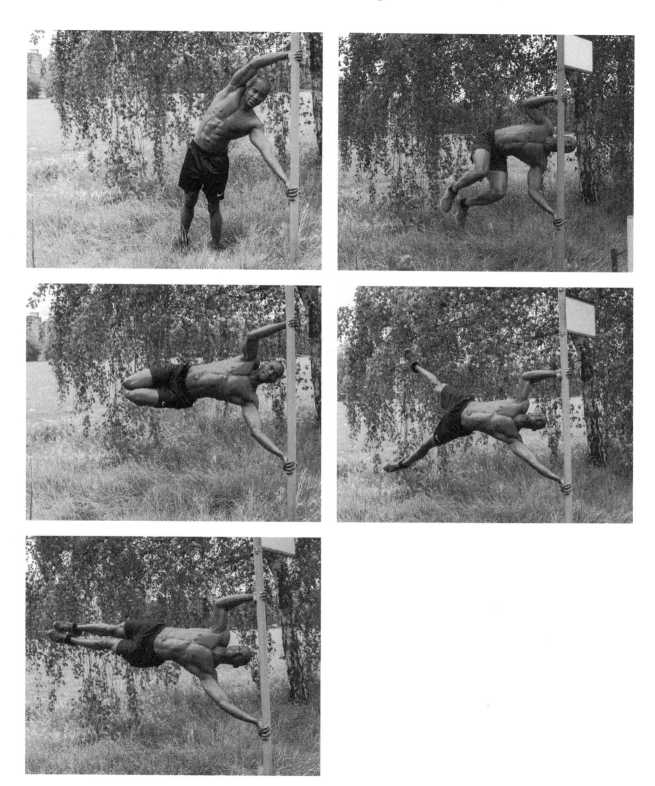

"Champions aren't made in gyms. Champions are made from something they have deep inside them — a desire, a dream, a vision. They have to have last-minute stamina, they have to be a little faster, they have to have the skill and the will. But the will must be stronger than the skill."

Muhammad Ali

6. CARDIO & CONDITIONING

Welcome to HELL! Your final task is to power through the fire and come out the other side keeled over, dripping in sweat, but completely and utterly satisfied that you left absolutely NOTHING on the table.

Yes, this is a book focused on calisthenics, but it would be criminal to omit cardiovascular exercise and general conditioning, as this is the gateway to a truly SUPERHUMAN body. By performing these exercises you will condition your body to be able to work harder and go longer, thereby allowing you to compound your results exponentially.

You will also turn your body into a fat burning furnace, blasting belly fat and allowing your finely tuned muscles to come to the fore. For building popping six-pack abs and obliques in particular, this is non-negotiable. We are truly into no pain, no gain territory!

Remember, the name of the game here is not slow and steady; conditioning is all about intensity. Throw everything you have at the following exercises – if your heart isn't pounding, if you're not covered in sweat, then you're not training hard enough!

Don't be one of those people who sits idly on a bike, scrolling through their Facebook feed and working out their thumbs more than the rest of their body. And you better not skip it altogether either, because this guide comes as a package, just like your body.

If you're still in doubt as to the benefits of cardio and conditioning, here's a quick recap:

1. INCREASE METABOLISM: This becomes increasingly important as the years go by and your metabolism slows down. In order to achieve a peak state of being, use cardio to keep your metabolism running at full throttle!

2. KEEP YOUR HEART HEALTHY: Your heart just so happens to be the muscle that runs the entire show, and cardiovascular exercise is how you give it a workout. Look after your ticker, and it will look after you!

3. IMPROVE RECOVERY TIME: A spot of cardio after a heavy session can reduce your DOMS (Delayed Onset of Muscle Soreness) and rush healing, oxygen rich blood to the muscle tissues. Translation: you can get back in the game quicker!

4. BURN FAT AND LOOK AWESOME: The simple fact of the matter is that you will never burn that stubborn fat and achieve your dream body without cardio. So, how about we just quit all this jibber jabber and knock it out of the park!

INTERVAL SPRINTS

Welcome to the pinnacle of cardio and conditioning exercises. Sprinting will get your heart pounding and your muscles working overtime to deliver INSANE results.

Super important: We must say it, but it truly is super important. Please, never perform cardiovascular activity without having had a thorough physical. Better safe than sorry.

Perform: 5-10 sets of 10-15 second bursts.

1. Take up the traditional starting position for a sprint, ready to spring off from one foot. If you are on a treadmill or free running, prepare to increase the speed.

2. With a powerful burst, break into as fast a sprint as you possibly can and do not stop until you reach your target to complete 1 set.

3. Rest for 30 secs or so and then go again. In this case, jogging can be a form of rest!

NB: Going from zero to everything can be risky, so make double sure that you have properly warmed up before launching into this kind of activity.

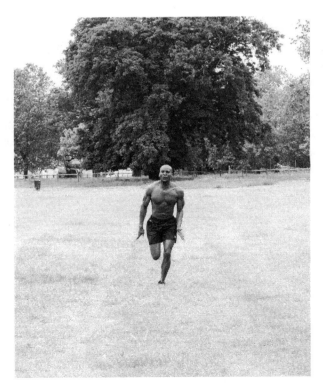
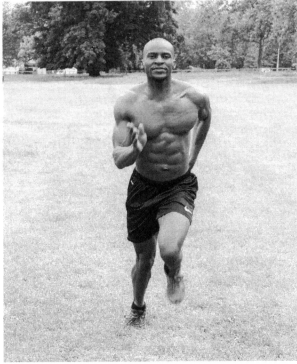

SKIPPING

Skipping is a great cardiovascular exercise that is often used for warming up or down as well as general fitness training.

Perform: 3-4 sets of 20-30 second bursts.

1. Grab your rope and swing it over your head.

2. From here you can either choose to jump both feet over the rope, or skip one foot at a time. If you're feeling really fancy, you can even do a criss cross.

Variation: Pick up a weighted rope for a greater challenge.

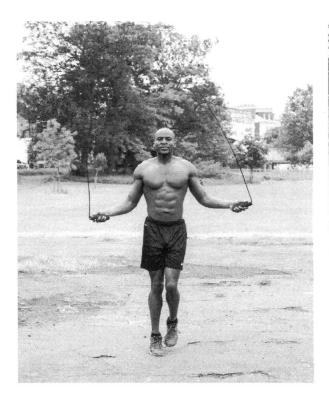
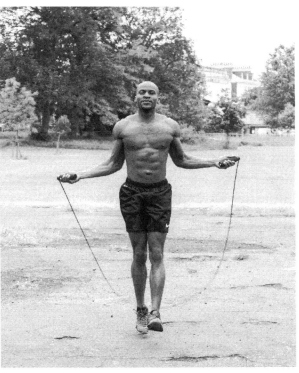

JUMPING SQUAT

We covered the squat earlier on so you should be used to performing this movement in some capacity already, but it's now time to explore a more intense alternative.

Perform: 3-4 sets of 20-30 reps.

1. Take up the same starting position as regular squats, standing with your feet shoulder width apart.

2. Squat down as you would for regular squats.

3. Launch yourself into the air as high as possible.

4. Upon landing, bend your knees to absorb the impact and compete one rep, using the momentum generated to launch straight into the next rep.

Remember: You can always mix things up by working out against the clock instead of using a sets and reps system.

A mixture of the two, i.e. seeing how may reps you can perform in a certain amount of time, can be particularly effective when training cardio.

It's useful to have a training buddy when it comes to this kind of exercise, as it is pretty darn exhausting and you might find their support helps you find the strength to rock out that final rep.

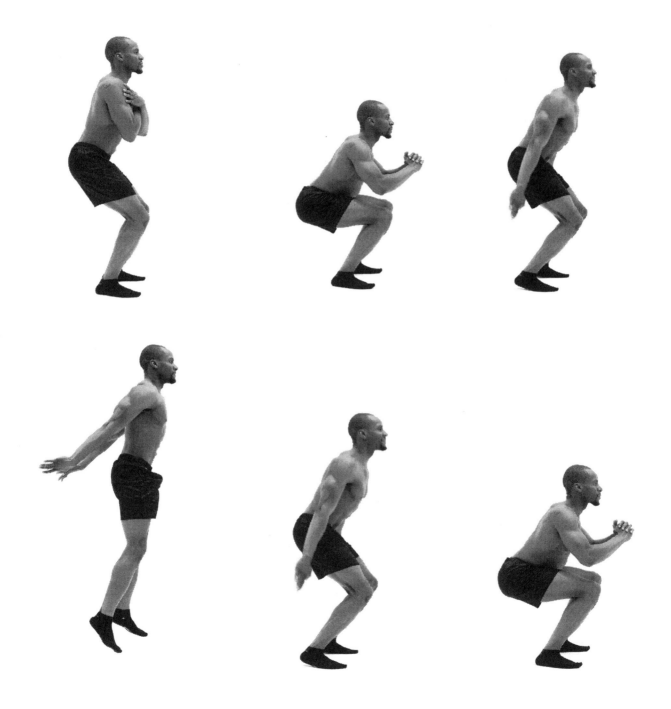

SQUAT THRUST

We're getting a little more advanced now, but most people should still be comfortable with this exercise, with a little practice.

You'll soon notice that you are also getting a pretty decent full body workout in addition to your cardio hit. Embrace it. It's all part of become your best self.

Perform: 3-4 sets of 20-30 reps.

1. Squat down on your toes with your knees tucked against your chest and palms flat on floor in front of your feet.

2. Keeping your palms rooted, spring your feet off the ground and propel them backwards so you effectively land in the push-up position.

3. Reverse the movement, springing your feet back into the starting position to complete one repetition.

NB: If you've just performed this exercise for the first time, you will realize that it's more than just a cardio hit.

The squat thrust also calls upon your arms for support, your lower body for that explosive push off, and above all your core for hauling yourself into position.

For those who straight up hate cardio, there is at least some solace to be had in the knowledge that you are working hard on those other key areas, too!

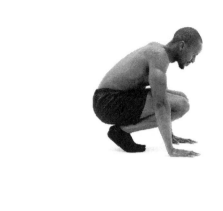

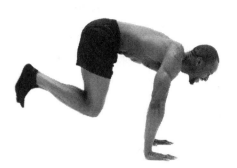

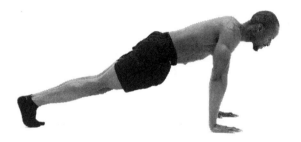

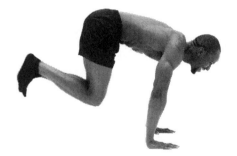

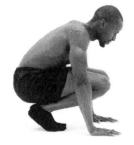

Mountain Climbers

Essentially a variation on the squat thrust, the mountain climber is an excellent addition to your cardio and conditioning repertoire.

Perform: 3-4 sets of 20-30 reps.

1. Take up the push-up position, except this time bring one foot right up until it's just behind your hands.

2. Spring your feet into the air and switch their positions, bringing the front one to the back and vice versa.

3. Reverse the action to bring your legs back to starting position to complete one rep. You can fire straight into the next rep from here.

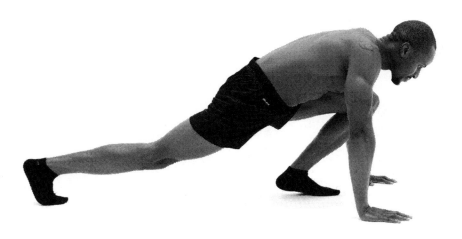

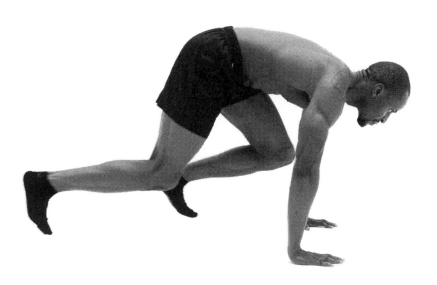

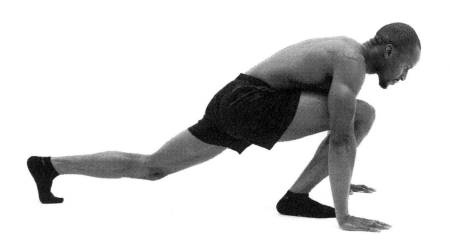

JUMPING LUNGE

Another variation on an exercise we've already covered, the jumping lunge is a great way to condition your lower body at the same time as getting an intense cardio hit.

Perform: 3-4 sets of 6-10 reps on each leg.

1. Take up the lunge position with one foot forward and both knees bent, the rear one close to the ground.

2. Jump into the air, aiming to get as much height as possible, and switch leg positions, bringing the front one to the back and vice versa.

3. Bend your knees upon landing to complete one repetition and use the momentum generated to go on and perform a full set.

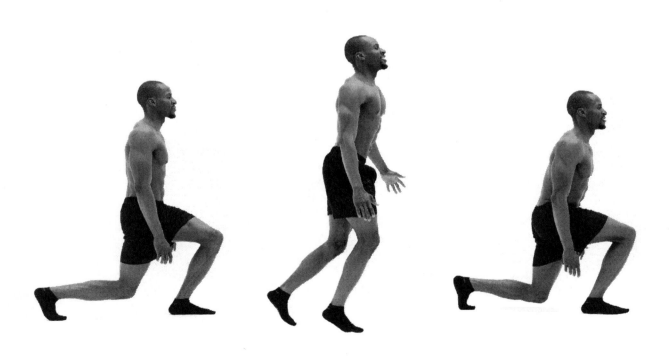

STAR JUMPS

Favored for its simplicity and famed for its effectiveness, the humble star jump is the staple of fitness regimes the world over. It is extremely likely that you have done this exercise before, but here's a reminder of how to complete it with proper form anyway.

Perform: 3-4 sets of 20-30 reps.

1. Stand up straight, feet together and arms by your sides.

2. Jump into the air stretching your arms and feet out to the sides.

3. Land with your feet wide apart and arms raised straight above your head.

4. Return to starting position by jumping up into the air again, bringing your feet back together and arms to your sides. You have now performed one repetition.

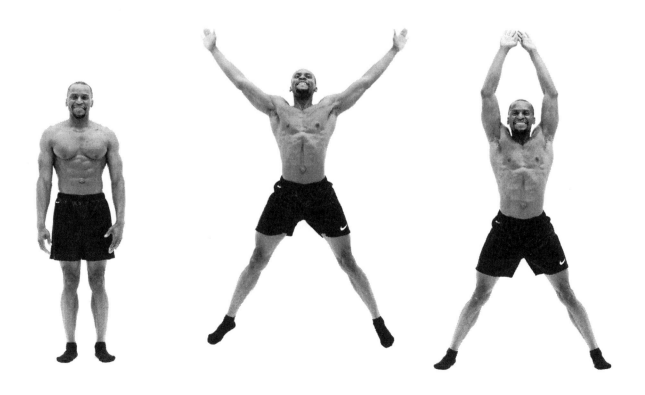

BURPEES

You are about to call upon every muscle sinew in your body to complete one of the most effective conditioning exercises known to man, so get warmed up and prepare for pain!

Perform: 3-4 sets of 10-20 reps.

1. Take up the squat thrust position, crouched down on your toes with your knees tucked against your chest and palms flat on floor in front of your feet.

2. Palms rooted, spring your feet into the air and thrust your legs backwards so you land in the push-up position.

3. Reverse this movement, springing your feet into the air again and landing back in the starting position.

4. Jump straight upwards as high as you can, bending your knees upon landing to again assume the position in step 1 to complete one rep.

Remember: Keep it moving with exercises like this. Pushing on through exhaustion is how progress is made. Never just go through the motions or quit as soon as the going gets tough!

You may find it particularly difficult to keep track of sets and reps when your heart is busy pumping oxygen to every extremity, so setting a timer and working to the clock is a great way to train if you're going solo.

If you have a training partner, have them count you down, and don't be afraid of a little competition. You might just bring the best out of each other.

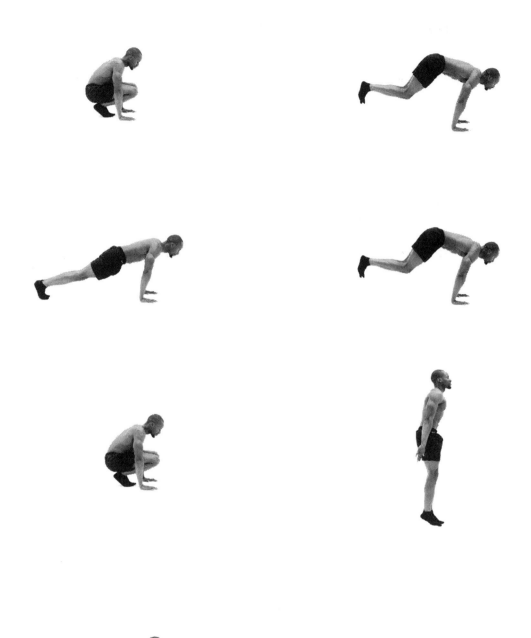

ADVANCED BURPEES

Essentially the same as the burpee, except we're tossing a push-up into the middle of each rep. Some call it the 'bastard', and you're about to find out why!

Perform: 3-4 sets of 10-20 reps.

1. Assume the same starting position as the burpee, crouched down, knees just behind your hands, braced for the punishment to come.

2. Now kick your feet back to push-up position as before.

3. Knock out 1 push-up.

4. When you are back at the top of the push-up position, kick your feet back to the crouched position.

5. Now jump straight up into the air, aiming for the moon!

6. Land back in the crouched position and go again.

Are you feeling the burn? If you said no, you're lying. But fear not, for we are about to draw this cardio and conditioning section to a close.

We have one more offering which is sure to attract some double takes out in public, but don't be afraid to go all in. After all, you get out exactly what you put in.

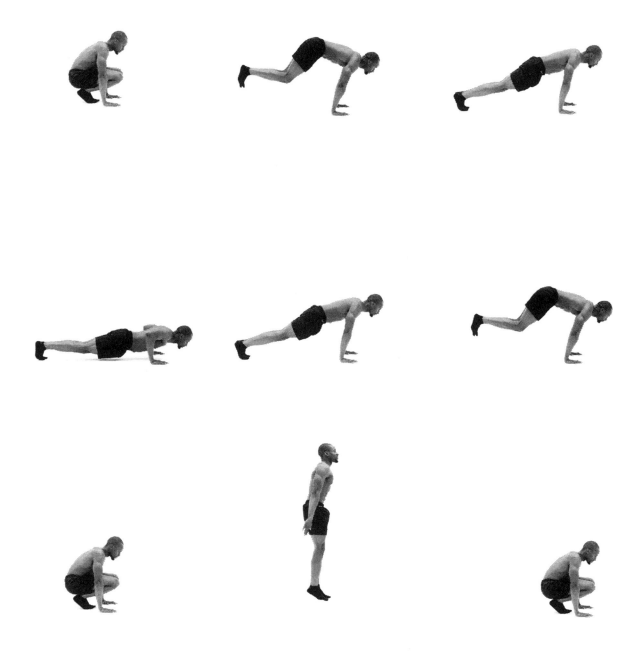

BEAR CRAWLS

This is another brutal conditioning exercise, but pain really does mean gain here so commit to completing it and you will see and feel the benefits.

Perform: 3-4 sets of 15-20 second crawls.

1. Take up the push-up position.

2. Place one hand forward, and bring the opposite foot forward too. Continue crawling like this, alternating your hands and legs, until you reach your threshold.

3. Repeat for allocated number of sets.

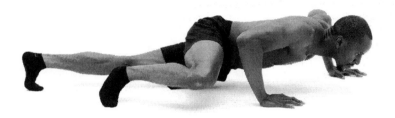

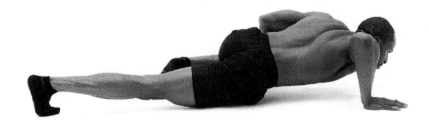

OTHER

You can probably see a trend building with cardio and conditioning – intense bursts of activity, followed by a short rest before going in all over again.

Cycling, rowing, boxing, circuits, swimming etc. are other great ways to get the blood pumping so don't be afraid to throw your own interests and hobbies into the mix.

It is generally recommended to perform 30-60 minutes of cardio per day. In addition to the benefits you already know of, you may also experience a myriad of other pros. These include reduced stress and anxiety, clarity of thought, improved sleep and even a potent antidote to depression. It really pays, then, to find a way to get your fix.

So long as your heart is pounding and your brow is dripping, you are doing cardio. It doesn't have to be by the book, but it does have to be done, and it does have to be tough. That is non-negotiable for those seeking SUPERHUMAN status.

Our mantra is simple: train hard. Two words that need to be etched into your mind whenever you enter the field of battle. Do not turn up to participate, turn up to WIN!

If you are training solo, every day should be an endeavor to reach a personal best or achieve something new. If you have a training buddy, push each other to higher levels by competing on every exercise. You will be shocked at just how far this takes you.

So, with that final gut-busting burst of activity we conclude this complete rundown of calisthenics exercises. You now possess the very same knowledge as the elite.

You have witnessed the unparalleled power of bodyweight exercise, and you have step-by-step instructions to achieve the body of your dreams.

Depending on your current level of ability, you may be ready to dive in at the deep end, or you might have to flip right back to the beginning and start at square one.

Our one key piece of advice is to understand and accept your level, and progress at your own pace. It is far more beneficial to make steady progress with proper form than it is to rush ahead and completely fail to achieve your objectives.

Flip the page for more advice on progressing with calisthenics.

7. Progressing With Calisthenics

Like any form of exercise it is essential to nail down the basics before progressing. In fact, the same is true of anything in life. As the old saying goes, walk before you can run!

You might be tempted to dive straight into a handstand or attempt a human flag but without sufficient practice you will not possess the strength or technique required in order to perform more advanced exercises.

Before you attempt something new, ask yourself one simple question and commit to answering truthfully: 'have I completed each number of sets or the hold time allocated for the easier exercises in this book absolutely perfectly?'

If the answer is 'no', then revisit the areas you still need to work on. By doing this you will gradually build a body that is properly prepared for advanced bodyweight exercises.

To help you reach that level in the fastest possible time, we've put together a beginner's calisthenics routine for you absolutely free. See the next page to get your copy now.

Once you have surpassed the beginner's level, or if you are already at intermediate or advanced capability, there is still plenty of room for improvement.

Arguably the greatest thing about calisthenics is that the possibilities are almost endless when it comes to inventing variations on established exercises, which means progress never stops, unless you do!

Once you can perform a base exercise, and have mastered each variation thereof, feel free to experiment with your own interpretations. So long as you maintain proper form, you will continue to experience phenomenal growth.

It is at this stage, when you are mastering high level exercises and coming up with your own innovative variations, that you can truly claim SUPERHUMAN status! To get there faster, join us at purecalisthenics.com for more resources.

You can also find the rest of the books in this series by searching 'Pure Calisthenics' on Amazon. In the meantime, get on a training program and go hard!

See you at SUPERHUMAN!

The Pure Calisthenics Team

8. BONUS: FREE TRAINING PROGRAM

You've got the exercises, now get the program! Download your bodyweight training routine free now and get on the road to total body perfection.

Here at Pure Calisthenics we're all about progressive teaching, and that is exactly what this program has been designed to achieve.

Build a solid foundation with this fundamental calisthenics routine, broken down into a full week of exercises, complete with suggested sets and reps.

Don't leave your results to chance; follow a proven program and take your first steps on the road to SUPERHUMAN right now!

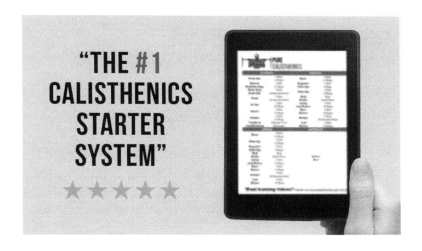

Visit www.purecalisthenics.com for your free program!

LIKE THIS BOOK?

The calisthenics community is all about sharing ideas and growing together. With that in mind, here's a few ways you can get involved:

1. If you got value from this book, or the free bonus training program, we'd be super stoked if you could head on over to your Amazon purchase history to leave a review.

2. The most powerful way to boost your progress is to share your journey with a friend. Put a call out on Facebook and Twitter, share this guide with a training partner and go crush it together!

3. To see our other books and resources, search 'Pure Calisthenics' on Amazon and visit www.purecalisthenics.com for bodyweight training tips, equipment reviews, nutrition advice and more!

So, all that remains to say is thanks for picking up this book. Don't forget to grab your free program and, as always, train hard!

The Pure Calisthenics Team

Review Now!

Share on Twitter

Share on Facebook

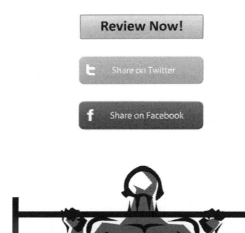

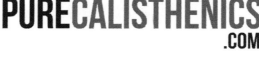

Made in the USA
Coppell, TX
24 June 2021